Evidence-based Practice for Nurses and Allied Health Professionals

5TH EDITION

Evidence-based Practice for Nurses and Allied Health Professionals

PAUL LINSLEY
ROS KANE

FOREWORD BY
JANET BARKER

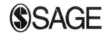

Los Angeles | London | New Delhi
Singapore | Washington DC | Melbourne

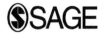

Los Angeles | London | New Delhi
Singapore | Washington DC | Melbourne

SAGE Publications Ltd
1 Oliver's Yard
55 City Road
London EC1Y 1SP

SAGE Publications Inc.
2455 Teller Road
Thousand Oaks, California 91320

SAGE Publications India Pvt Ltd
B 1/I 1 Mohan Cooperative Industrial Area
Mathura Road
New Delhi 110 044

SAGE Publications Asia-Pacific Pte Ltd
3 Church Street
#10-04 Samsung Hub
Singapore 049483

Editor: Alex Clabburn
Assistant editor: Ruth Lily
Production editor: Sarah Sewell
Copyeditor: Jane Fricker
Proofreader: Clare Weaver
Indexer: Melanie Gee
Marketing manager: Ruslana Khatagova
Cover design: Sheila Tong
Typeset by: C&M Digitals (P) Ltd, Chennai, India
Printed in the UK

Library of Congress Control Number: 2021949253

British Library Cataloguing in Publication data

A catalogue record for this book is available from the
British Library

ISBN 978-1-5297-7592-1
ISBN 978-1-5297-7591-4 (pbk)

At SAGE we take sustainability seriously. Most of our products are printed in the UK using responsibly sourced
papers and boards. When we print overseas we ensure sustainable papers are used as measured by the PREPS
grading system. We undertake an annual audit to monitor our sustainability.

Contents

About the Editors and Contributors

ABOUT THE FOUNDING AUTHOR

Dr Janet Barker was the original author of this book. She was involved in nursing for over 40 years, starting as a cadet nurse at 16 years of age in an orthopaedic hospital, moving into general nursing and finally working as a mental health nurse, in both inpatient and community settings. The last 20 years of her career were spent in nurse education. Janet has vast experience of organising and delivering undergraduate pre-registration nursing courses, taking on the role of Course Director of the Diploma/BSc (Hons) in Nursing programme at the University of Nottingham, School of Nursing, Midwifery and Physiotherapy in 2005. Janet received the University of Nottingham 'Dearing Award' in 2011 in recognition of her 'outstanding contribution to the development of teaching and student learning'. She retired as Associate Professor at the University of Nottingham in July 2011, however continues to keep abreast of current developments in nursing.

ABOUT THE EDITORS

Dr Paul Linsley has worked largely in acute and forensic mental health settings both as a clinician and as a manager. He is registered as a clinical specialist in Acute Psychiatry and is trained in Cognitive Behavioural Therapy.

As an Associate Professor of Nursing for the University of East Anglia he teaches on a number of courses, both single and joint honours undergraduate programmes, research masters programmes and pre- and post-registration specialist programmes. He supervises doctoral students and sits on several interest panels and committees.

Paul has worked on a number of research projects both as part of a team and as Principal Investigator, mainly around his interest of acute and forensic mental health. He has also undertaken commission work for the Welsh Assembly and Scottish Health Board. Paul has presented at international conferences and holds a number of awards. He is the author of several textbooks on nursing and health-related matters, one of which has been translated into Arabic and one into Japanese. Paul has an interest in values-based practice and this is reflected in his work both as a clinician and academic.

Dr Ros Kane is an Associate Professor and Director of Research in the School of Health and Social Care at the University of Lincoln in England where she co-leads the Mental Health, Health and Social Care Research Group (MH2aSC). She is also a Visiting Professor at Suratthani Rajahbat University in Thailand. With a background in nursing, Ros later graduated from University College London (UCL) with a BSc (Hons) in Anthropology and Geography and from the London School of Hygiene and Tropical Medicine (LSHTM) with an MSc in Medical Demography. Ros worked for 10 years in the Centre for Sexual and Reproductive Health Research at LSHTM where she completed her PhD in 2005 (a study into the optimal provision of sexual health services for young people in England). She has a strong interest in quality improvement as well as service and policy evaluation, particularly in relation to Public Health. Ros is the lead for the National Institute for Health Research/Health Education England's Integrated Clinical Academic Careers Internship Programme, a pre-masters research programme for nurses, midwives and allied health professionals across the East Midlands region in England.

ABOUT THE CONTRIBUTORS

Dr Christine Jackson has a background in Radiotherapy and Oncology where she has worked in both clinical and academic environments. Her PhD relates to assessment of clinical competence in the newly qualified radiotherapy workforce. She has worked at the University of Nottingham in England as a multi-professional advisor for the Postgraduate Medical Deanery and the Trent Workforce Development Confederation. She has also worked in partnership with the Department of Health on a number of projects including the StLaR HR Plan Project and the UKCRC subcommittee for nurses in Clinical Research. Christine was instrumental in working with Professor Tony Butterworth to establish the national framework for Clinical Academic Careers. She moved to the University of Lincoln in 2005 and led on the development of Clinical Academic Career Training. Christine is also a Visiting Professor at the University of Maribor in Slovenia and is co-founder and first chair of the international UDINE-C network (Understanding Development Issues in Nurse Educator Careers).

Dr David Nelson is a Research Fellow in Rural Health and Care within the Lincoln International Institute for Rural Health (LIIRH) in the College of Social Science, the University of Lincoln. In addition to his role with LIIRH, David is a registered Macmillan Cancer Support Professional and prior to this, worked as a Research Assistant in the School of Health and Social Care at the University of Lincoln (2014–15), and in the School of Government and Public Policy, at the University of Strathclyde in Glasgow (2013). He currently holds professional membership of the Social Research Association (SRA) and the Scottish Rural Health Partnership (SRHP). His primary research interests are in the field of cancer survivorship – in particular, the role of rural–urban residency and how this impacts on health behaviours and self-management following cancer treatment, which was the focus of his mixed methods PhD.

Marishona Ortega is a Chartered Librarian and has worked in the field of health and medical librarianship for 20 years both within the NHS and the academic sectors. Her professional interests include literature searching and evidence retrieval, systematic reviews and critical appraisal. She is a Fellow of the Higher Education Academy and is currently Senior Academic Subject Librarian: Bio-Medicine & Health Sciences at the University of Lincoln.

Karen Johnston is a registered mental health nurse with a range of experience in clinical services, workforce planning and education commissioning as part of Health Education England. Karen is a Senior Lecturer in Mental Health Nursing with the University of Lincoln in the UK having worked as a Matron for Safe Staffing and Professional Development within a mental health trust before joining the University. Karen's specialisms include workforce planning and transformation, and health service commissioning. Karen is also a practising hypnotherapist.

Foreword

When I first considered writing a book on Evidence Based Practice (EBP) in 2007, the concept was a relatively new, but essential element of healthcare delivery. At that time, I was working in nurse education, teaching the principles of EBP not only to pre- and post-registration students at undergraduate level but also to those undertaking post-graduate courses. I was aware that the undergraduate students were often overwhelmed by the volume of information they were expected to assimilate, finding the language of some aspects strange and incomprehensible. Post-graduate students, having grasped the basic underpinnings, needed an easily accessible synopsis of EBP, something to act as a reminder when trying to integrate the concepts into their busy, everyday working lives of clinical practice. My aim, therefore, was to provide a useful aid to practitioners, something which explored the nature and underpinning theory of EBP, supporting its implementation in a clear and understandable way. I wanted to provide a step-by-step guide for novice nurses, giving them access to key concepts of EBP and tools that would facilitate its implementation. Equally, my intention was to produce a source of materials to assist experienced practitioners in their day-to-day practice. This remained at the heart of the book in all its iterations, as it grew to address the needs of a wider range of healthcare professionals.

I had little idea when the first edition was published that, over 10 years later, a fifth edition would be a reality. I am immensely proud and pleased to write the foreword for this latest publication. Both the co-editors, Paul Linsley and Ros Kane, have vast knowledge, experience and expertise in their chosen professional fields. I had the pleasure of working with Paul in nurse education for a number of years. Ros, I came to know and respect whilst collaborating with her in the writing of the book's third edition. They have both added to, and enhanced the nature and scope of the book, enabling it to evolve into something which has proven useful and insightful to practitioners of today and tomorrow.

EBP is now firmly established as key to the development and sustainability of high quality care; however, it remains a complex activity. The rapidly changing face of healthcare has resulted in the development of new ways of working. This required the introduction of practice development; improvement and innovation initiatives to enable practitioners to adapt to and integrate new approaches into their sphere of practice. To enable healthcare to move forward there has been a need to find ways to encourage continuous personal and professional development. The growing belief in the centrality of patient/service user and carer involvement in the decision making and delivery of care has resulted in an expansion of the approaches and tools available to facilitate such activities. The various editions of this book chart these developments in healthcare theory and practice over the last 10 years, with each new revision incorporating and expanding on the predominant issues facing the modern practitioner at that time.

The fifth edition remains true to the underpinning and founding principles of the original book, providing a resource that is current, accessible and useful to a range of practitioners and students. The editors, Paul and Ros, carry the book forward in an insightful and authoritative way, offering an essential guide to all aspects of EBP, whilst, at the same time, providing tools and resources which will prove invaluable to the practitioners in modern healthcare settings. Therefore, it is with the greatest confidence that I commend this fifth edition of *Evidence-based Practice for Nurses and Allied Health Professionals* to you, the reader.

Preface

Welcome to the fifth edition of *Evidence-based Practice for Nurses and Allied Health Professionals*. The book is an essential resource for students and staff and highlights the importance of providing clinical practice based on sound evidence. It provides a clear and measured account of the increasing need for clinicians to be able to articulate the knowledge on which they make decisions and the part that evidence plays in driving practice forward. To practise effectively, nurses and other healthcare professionals need to be able to discern between the different sources of evidence available to them in order to make the best possible decisions in the interest of the patient at the time required. In order to do this, they need to be able to critically evaluate the evidence presented and make use of this in an informed way. This book explores the concept of evidence-based practice through a number of different lenses and provides practical guidance on its utilisation in clinical practice. The book has been revised to ensure that it remains contemporary and includes the provision of a chapter on the history and development of clinical academic careers which are becoming increasingly embedded across the educational and clinical sectors.

There are a number of ways in which this book can be used. Those new to the concept of evidence-based practice may want to work through the chapters chronologically to gain the necessary knowledge and skills in a step-by-step way. Those with some existing understanding may want use individual chapters as a point of reference, according to learning need. The book has also been written to support academic health and social care curricula and is a useful educational resource for a number of disciplines. Each chapter begins with a list of learning outcomes and ends with a summary of the main points, suggestions for further reading and useful weblinks. Key terms are highlighted, and definitions given in the glossary.

WHAT'S IN THE BOOK?

The book falls into three parts. Part I examines the key elements of evidence-based practice. Chapter 1 considers what EBP is and why it is important that practitioners understand and develop the necessary knowledge and skills to deliver it. Chapter 2 explores issues in relation to the nature of knowledge and where it comes from; what knowledge is seen as underpinning clinical practice; what counts as good and appropriate evidence. It also introduces important concepts pertaining to gaining appropriate ethical and governance approvals when conducting clinical research. Chapter 3 considers issues related to clinical judgement, expertise and decision making. Chapter 4 discusses how to locate evidence and develop a search strategy and is very practical in its approach.

Part II provides an opportunity to explore the knowledge and skills associated with the critical appraisal of evidence, beginning with Chapter 5, which identifies what is meant by critical appraisal and its role in the EBP process. Chapters 6 and 7 look at critical appraisal specifically in relation to quantitative and qualitative research respectively. Chapter 8 considers issues related to systematic review and its place in evidence-based practice. Critical appraisal tools to help with this process are provided in the appendices.

Finally, Part III looks at how to make changes to practice once appropriate evidence has been identified and critically appraised. Chapter 9 discusses the differences between health service evaluation, audit and research. At times the distinction between the three can be blurred and confusing. However, there are distinct differences in the evidence they produce and the way in which the evidence is used by clinicians and managers as part of clinical practice. Chapter 10 considers how evidence is used to shape and change practice as part of practice development, improvement and innovation. Chapter 11 examines the development of clinical academic careers and their impact on clinical practice and benefits for nurses, midwives and allied healthcare professionals.

The editors hope you will find the book a useful resource, one that helps you to develop the knowledge and skills needed to ensure patients receive the best care possible – based on good evidence, aimed at achieving positive outcomes.

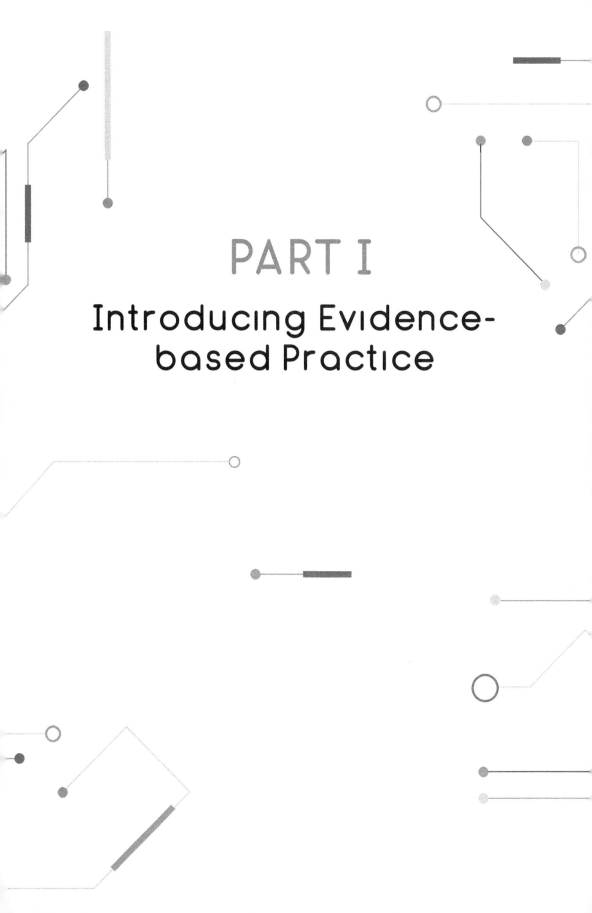

PART I
Introducing Evidence-based Practice

1

Introduction: What is Evidence-based Practice?

Paul Linsley and Ros Kane

Learning Outcomes

By the end of the chapter, you will be able to:

- define evidence-based practice;
- understand how evidence-based practice came into being;
- discuss the pros and cons of evidence-based practice;
- identify the components of evidence-based practice and the skills associated with it;
- consider why your practice needs to be evidence-based.

INTRODUCTION

Since its introduction in the 1990s Evidence-based Practice (EBP) has had a direct impact on health and social care policy the world over. The COVID-19 pandemic has been a poignant reminder of the importance of EBP and how much it informs and shapes our clinical practice. The pandemic has led to a surge of information being presented to clinicians and has shaped the care and treatment people have received. As our understanding of the virus has grown so too has the **evidence** presented to clinicians and the public. One of the difficulties faced by clinicians has been discerning what is the best evidence on which to base their decisions. The acquisition of the skills needed to scrutinise and critique research evidence has therefore arguably never been more important to health professionals as it is today and provides the main focus for this book.

EBP is a global phenomenon which promotes the idea of best practice, clinical effectiveness and quality care and involves an integration of evidence, clinical expertise, patient preferences and the context of care delivery to inform clinical decision making. Government initiatives have promoted EBP as a way of providing both clinically effective and cost-effective healthcare and it has been used to pursue changes to clinical practice and healthcare systems. It provides clinicians with a method to critically appraise scientifically proven evidence for delivering quality healthcare to a specific population.

EBP is fundamental to the way in which nurses and other healthcare professionals approach their work, and in the decisions that they make. A nurse, like all other healthcare professionals, is primarily a knowledge worker. To practise effectively, healthcare professionals need to be able to discern between the different sources of evidence and information available to them in order to make the best possible decision in the interests of the patient at the time required. For nurses, this translates into combining clinical evidence, individual expertise and patient preferences with the goal of providing good quality care. Patients (and their families) expect the care we deliver to be evidence-based, and as healthcare professionals we are accountable for our actions – having an evidence base for those actions is therefore essential. We also know that evidence-based care improves patients' outcomes and lives. In the UK, it has been reported that research-active healthcare organisations have better outcomes, including survival (King's Fund, 2019).

But we also know that the evidence base changes over time, as does knowledge, and we need to keep up with those changes. The volume of existing evidence, and keeping up with new emerging evidence, can sometimes seem daunting. The amount of evidence is increasing year on year. Since the first randomised controlled trial in 1948, the number of trials has grown exponentially with around 150,000 published by 2004, and well over a million published today. Trials are just one form of evidence. There is also a mass of observational work and increasing numbers of systematic reviews and clinical guidelines. We need strategies to help us identify the relevant evidence from this myriad of sources, and we will show you how to do this as we go through the book.

While there are a number of definitions for EBP, perhaps the best known and accepted of these is that by Sackett et al. (1996), who defined it as:

> The conscientious, explicit, and judicious use of current best practice in making decisions about the care of individual patients. The practice of evidence-based medicine means integrating individual clinical experience with best available external clinical evidence from systematic research. (Sackett et al., 1996: 71)

This definition, while proving popular, has been criticised, as it seemingly ignores the contribution that patients play in the decision-making process. Muir Gray (1997) sought to address this shortfall in thinking by building on the work of Sackett and his team and put forward this definition in response:

> Evidence based practice is an approach to decision making in which the clinician uses the best evidence available, in consultation with the patient, to decide upon the option which suits the patient best. (Muir Gray, 1997: 3)

The above definition highlights the need to consult with the patient and involve them in decisions about their own health and wellbeing. It also takes into account patients' preferences, including their wish to avoid risks associated with interventions. Indeed, Sackett and his team (2000: 1) developed a simpler but more telling definition of EBP in response to Muir Gray's work, and defined EBP as: 'The integration of the best research evidence with clinical expertise and patient values'.

This notion of patient involvement is echoed in more contemporary definitions of EBP; for instance,

> [EBP] involves using the best evidence you have about the most effective care of individuals, using it with the person's best interests in mind, to the best of your ability and in such a way that it is clear to others that you are doing it. (Lindsay, 2007: 17)

EBP is important because healthcare is complex and there can be uncertainty in people's response to treatment and uncertainty in people's experiences of treatment. So, decision making in healthcare requires full consideration of the evidence. Implicit in such discussions is the message that healthcare, wherever it is delivered, must be based on good, sound evidence. It has been suggested that, historically, clinical issues have been based on a form of craft-based knowledge or 'habit, intuition and sometimes plain old guessing' (Gawande, 2003: 7). This is no longer sufficient and there is an expectation that strong evidence must underpin clinical practice. Indeed, healthcare professionals have a responsibility to practise evidence-based care, and this is reinforced in policy and clinical guidance the world over.

Reflect on the evidence that underpins your clinical practice. Where does this evidence come from? How do you keep up to date with current developments and changes in practice? How easy is it to make changes to your practice using new evidence?

Activity 1.1

While the importance of research in the delivery of care has always been emphasised, the idea of evidence-based practice is seen as focusing the minds of those involved in care delivery on the use of appropriate evidence. Healthcare professionals need to be certain that their practice is current and that they are doing the best for those that they look after. EBP provides them with the means by which to explore practice and address any shortfall in the care that they give. The question then becomes one of how can the evidence be located? With the advent of the internet, busy healthcare professionals can no longer hope to keep up to date with all the possible sources of evidence, nor can they read and critically appraise all of the articles relevant to their practice. This is why an evidence-based approach to practice is needed. EBP provides a systematic framework for reviewing the evidence to underpin practice. There is a range of such evidence that can inform practice – personal experience and **reflection**, literature, research, policy, guidelines, clinical expertise and audit (Dale, 2005) – all of which have their place within EBP and will be explored further in the various chapters of this book.

WHERE DID THE IDEA OF EBP COME FROM?

Professor Archie Cochrane, a British epidemiologist, is most frequently credited with start-ing the EBP movement. In his book *Effectiveness and Efficiency: Random Reflections on the Health Service* (Cochrane, 1972) he criticised the medical profession for not using appropri-ate evidence to guide and direct medical practice and challenged medicine to produce an evidence base. He argued there was a need to ensure treatment was delivered in the most effective manner and to ensure that available evidence was used in a consistent way.

When Cochrane talked of evidence, he meant randomised control trials (RCTs), which he viewed as providing the most reliable evidence on which to base medical care. RCTs are a form of research that use experimental designs to identify the effectiveness of interventions. The use of systematic reviews, which summarise the findings of a number of RCTs looking at similar areas of interest, was suggested as the 'gold standard' of the scientific evidence on which to base medical interventions.

The medical profession responded to Cochrane's challenge by creating the Cochrane Centre for systematic reviews, which opened in 1992 in Oxford. The Cochrane Collaboration was founded in 1993, consisting of international review groups (currently encompassing more than 28,000 people in over 100 countries) covering a range of clinical areas and producing systematic reviews. These reviews are published electronically, updated regularly and there are now over 4,600 available.

Activity 1.2

Visit the Cochrane Collaboration website (www.cochrane.org). How easy is the site to navigate? What sort of evidence does the site provide? How useful is the evidence? Could you readily relate to/make use of this evidence as part of your clinical practice?

While the underpinning principles of **evidence-based medicine** (EBM) were hotly debated, the medical profession in general began to accept the idea, and 1995 saw the first issue of the journal *Evidence-Based Medicine for Primary Care and Internal Medicine*, published by the British Medical Journal Group. In 2007 EBM was identified as one of 15 major milestones in the development of medical practice since 1840 (*BMJ*, 2007). Nursing, emulating its medical counterpart, began to explore the notion of basing its practice on reliable sources of evidence, which resulted in the journal *Evidence-Based Nursing*, first published in 1998.

It has been argued, rightly so, that Florence Nightingale was also a pioneer of EBP. During the Crimean War, wounded British troops were shipped across the Black Sea to hospitals in Turkey. Nightingale arrived in Turkey in October 1854 with a group of vol-untary nurses. Initially they were denied entry to the hospital wards – it was not until the hospitals had reached a critical state in March 1855 that she and her nurses were allowed proper access to the patients. She realised that soldiers would die needlessly from malnu-trition, poor sanitation, and lack of activity, and she strove to improve living conditions,

keeping meticulous records of the death toll in the hospitals as evidence of the importance of patient welfare. She created graphs to highlight the death toll and its causes, and
crucially the collection, analysis, interpretation and presentation of this evidence led to a
change in practice.

SOCIAL AND POLITICAL DRIVERS OF EBP

Scott and McSherry (2008) suggested a number of social and political factors that facilitated
the emergence of the emphasis on evidence. The availability of 'knowledge' via the internet
and other sources brought into being 'expert patients' – well-educated and informed individuals who accessed information relating to health and illness. The expectations of these expert
patients were that healthcare professions would be aware of and use up-to-date information/
research in their delivery of care and treatment. There was no longer a willingness simply to
accept treatment or care purely on the advice of a doctor or nurse.

　The concept of EBP was also seen as attractive by governments and health service
administrators because of its potential to provide cost-effective and clinically effective
care (McSherry et al., 2006). In the mid-1990s the UK government of the day identified that quality assurance was to be placed at the forefront of the NHS modernisation
agenda. Two White Papers – *The New NHS: Modern and Dependable* (Department of
Health [DH], 1997) and *A First Class Service: Quality in the New NHS* (DH, 1998) –
outlined the plans for promoting **clinical effectiveness** and introducing **clinical
governance**. These promoted systems to ensure quality improvement mechanisms
were adopted at all levels of healthcare provision. Central to clinical governance were
concepts of risk management and promoting clinical excellence. (See Figure 1.1 for an
outline of the clinical governance framework.)

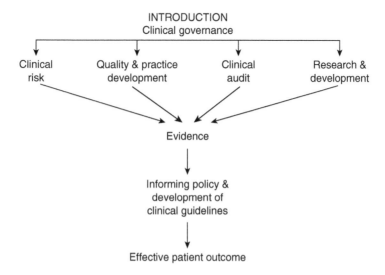

Figure 1.1　Representation of the elements of clinical governance

Clinical effectiveness was defined by the NHS Executive (1996) as 'the extent to which specific clinical interventions when deployed in the field for a particular patient or population, do what they are intended to do, that is maintain and improve health and secure the greatest possible health gain'. This definition continued to underpin the more recent Department of Health approach to clinical effectiveness (DH, 2007), with the various stages of the process being identified as:

- the development of best practice guidelines;
- the transfer of knowledge into practice through education, audit and practice development;
- the evaluation of the impact of guidelines through audit and patient feedback.

Put simply, clinical effectiveness can be seen as identifying appropriate evidence in the form of research, clinical guidelines, systematic reviews and national standards; changing practice to include this evidence; and evaluating the impact of any change and making the necessary adjustments through the use of **clinical audit** and patient feedback/**service evaluation**. Reading and understanding research, being aware of current policies and procedures, and knowing about the recommendations and standards in practice are all part of the nurse's role (Royal College of Nursing, 2007).

Two organisations were created in order to promote an evidence-based approach to healthcare, which are known today as the National Institute for Health and Care Excellence (NICE) and the Care Quality Commission (CQC). These bodies provide guidance for healthcare managers and practitioners and were charged with ensuring this guidance was followed in England and Wales. In Scotland the Health Technology Board fulfilled a similar purpose. Clinical governance was introduced to ensure healthcare was both efficient and effective; healthcare professionals were expected to show EBP supported all aspects of care delivery and service developments. It was hoped that the introduction of these measures would result in a shift in organisational culture from one that was reactive, responding as issues arise, to one with a proactive ethos, where the healthcare offered was known to be effective and, therefore, avoided unforeseen outcomes.

NICE and the CQC have continued to develop strategies to promote clinical effectiveness; the former through initiatives such as 'How to...' guides, quality standards and supporting a resource known as 'NHS Evidence'. The NHS Evidence website provides access to various forms of evidence that may be of use in clinical practice and provides examples of best practice. The CQC was charged with ensuring the safety and quality of care through inspection and assessment of all healthcare provision. The NHS Institute for Innovation and Improvement was set up in 2006 with a remit to support the implementation of service improvement initiatives within the NHS (although this was subsequently dissolved).

Activity 1.3

Identify one condition/disease you have come across recently in clinical practice. Visit the NICE website (www.nice.org.uk) and locate the NICE guidance and NHS evidence available in relation to your chosen condition/disease. Now ask the same questions you did of the Cochrane database: How easy is the site to navigate? What sort of evidence does the site provide? How useful is the evidence? Could you readily relate to/make use of this evidence as part of your clinical practice?

WHY DOES YOUR PRACTICE NEED TO BE EVIDENCE-BASED?

The need for frontline staff to be empowered to deliver a quality service is a major aspect of contemporary healthcare policy. As Craig and Stevens (2011) have already identified, few would disagree with the ideas underpinning EBP – namely, that care should be of the highest standard and delivered in the most effective way. Indeed, practising without any 'evidence' to guide actions amounts to little more than providing care that is based on trial and error, which would not be advocated. However, as identified above, care is not always based on the best evidence, with Greenhalgh (2014) suggesting that many of the decisions made in healthcare are based on four main sources of information:

1. *Anecdotal information.* Here it is considered that 'it worked in situation X so it must be appropriate to (the similar) situation Y'. However, as Greenhalgh points out, while situations may seem very similar, patient responses are often very different.
2. *Press cuttings information.* Here changes are made to practice in response to reading one article or editorial, without critically appraising and considering the applicability of those results to the specific setting.
3. *Consensus statements.* Here a group of 'experts' will identify the best approaches based on their experiences/beliefs. While clinical expertise does have a place in EBP, it does not operate without some problems. For example, clinical wisdom once held (and to a certain extent still does hold) that bed rest was the most appropriate form of treatment for acute lower back pain. However, research in 1986 demonstrated that this is potentially harmful.
4. *Cost minimisation.* Here the limited resources available within a healthcare setting will often result in choosing the cheapest option in an effort to spread resources as widely as possible. However, EBP can ensure the most effective use of limited and pressurised resources. While certain types of care may appear more expensive on the surface, if these prove more effective, they may turn out to be cheaper in the long run.

So, what is good evidence? What should we be using to inform our decision making? Well, we need to use research, but not just any research: it needs to be research that answers clinically relevant questions – so research that finds answers to questions that might inform our practice – and it needs to be research that has been robustly designed and conducted. In order to engage with, understand, and evaluate research, healthcare professionals need to understand what research is, how it is done, what good research looks like, and to see its applicability to their clinical practice.

Despite widespread recognition of the need for clinical practice to be based on sound evidence, frontline staff experience considerable challenges in implementing evidence-based care at an individual and organisational level. In particular, frontline nurses have difficulty interpreting research findings, and although willing to use research they often lack the skills to do so. Perhaps part of the problem related to nursing developing an EBP ethos is that it is often considered as more of an art than a science, and, as such, certain types of evidence are valued above others, such as expert opinion and practice experience. The complexities of healthcare, and the uncertainty of people's responses to and experiences of different types of interventions, require that full consideration is given to all available evidence.

Patients are likely to know a great deal about their own health needs and to expect health professionals to base care decisions on the most up-to-date and clinically relevant information. There is also an expectation that professionals will be able to comment in an informed way on any research reported in the media and identify its relevance to an individual's health needs. Miller and Forrest (2001) proposed that the ability to ensure that professionals' knowledge and skills remain current increases their professional credibility; allows them to be an important source of information to those in their care as well as colleagues; and enables all professionals involved in care delivery to make well-informed decisions. It has also been suggested that EBP can foster a **lifelong learning** approach – an essential requirement in the health professions if staff are to remain effective in rapidly changing healthcare environments (see Figure 1.2).

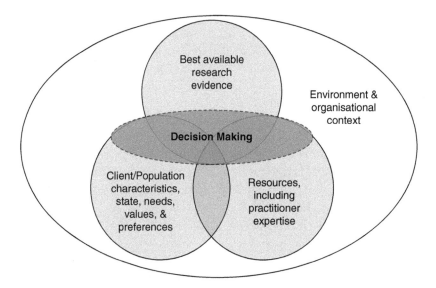

Figure 1.2   The integrated elements of EBP

Source: Council for Training in Evidence-Based Behavioural Practice (2008).

CONCERNS ABOUT EBP

Evidence-based approaches are not without their problems. As Wilkinson et al. (2011: 8) identified, EBP has both 'enthusiastic supporters and vociferous detractors'. Melnyk and Fineout-Overholt (2018) suggest that EBP is viewed by many as simply another term for research utilisation. It has also been argued elsewhere that the value of research has been over-emphasised to the detriment of clinical judgement and person-centred approaches, while others point to a lack of evidence to support the notion that EBP improves health outcomes.

Kitson (2002) has pointed to an inherent tension between EBP and person-centred approaches. She has argued that clinical expertise is vital in ensuring that patients' experiences and needs are not sidelined in the pursuit of 'best evidence' in the form of research findings and the development of generalised clinical guidelines. Some individuals have suggested that such broad general principles are not applicable to certain aspects of care. Wilkinson et al. (2011) suggested that practitioners often feel that an over-emphasis on EBP inhibits their ability to provide individualised care. Melnyk and Fineout-Overholt (2018) have identified this as a 'cookbook' approach, where a general recipe is followed with no consideration for the specific needs or preferences of individuals. There are concerns also around the ability to reach a consensus in relation to the various interpretations available when translating evidence into guidelines and the relevance of these for individual areas of practice. There are also issues related to the updating of evidence and the ability to ensure that the information gathered is current. However, DiCenso et al. (2013) argue that as clinical expertise and decision-making processes are central to EBP, in considering the use of general guidelines both of these processes must be used in the same way with any form of evidence including guidance.

Brady and Lewin (2007) argue that while the idea of clinical expertise is readily accepted by most experienced nurses, the majority of those same nurses are often unaware of the latest research in their area of practice. Nurses are generally presented as relying on intuition, tradition and local policies/procedures to guide their practice. There is also a perceived lack of enthusiasm in relation to the implementation of nursing research. Stevens (2013) proposed that healthcare providers frequently do not use current knowledge for a number of reasons, not least of these being the rapidly growing and changing body of research, some of which is difficult to apply to practice directly. As the aim of EBP is to deliver high-quality care, nurses need to have an understanding of what the exact elements of EBP are and to then develop the necessary skills and knowledge to enable them to carry this out. Glasziou and Haynes (2005) suggested that some research, essential to the delivery of quality care, will go unrecognised for years and suggested the major barriers to using evidence are time, effort and the skills involved in accessing information from the myriad of data available.

Ingersoll (2000) also argued that focusing EBP on care delivery reflects the differences between it and research. Research concentrates on knowledge discovery whereas in EBP the application of knowledge is central. In addition, she has suggested that while this emphasis on EBP is a welcome initiative, the wholesale 'lifting' of approaches and methodologies from another discipline such as medicine is not. Healthcare professionals need to make sure that the evidence used is relevant to their area of practice. There is a traditional view that evidence-based practice should be informed solely through quantitative research. However, Ellis (2010) advocates that it is more about using various forms of information, not just research, to guide and develop practice. Ellis (2010) goes on to note that there is little agreement between professionals as to what constitutes 'good evidence'. While nurses may be motivated to approach practice from an evidence-based perspective, the literature actually suggests that evidence-based practice is rigid and prescriptive, and diminishes any professional autonomy. French (1999) went further to suggest that as EBP is so closely linked with evidence-based medicine (EBM) and its preference for certain types of evidence, there is a danger that this promotes the use of medical knowledge over other forms and, therefore, leads to a medicalisation of healthcare environments to the detriment of other disciplines. Best evidence in the medical context is often taken to mean quantitative research findings in the form of RCTs. Some have questioned its compatibility with nursing and the other health professions, suggesting instead the use of a more open approach. Dale (2005) proposed that this issue has the potential to create interprofessional conflict, as that which nursing may count as appropriate evidence on which to base practice may be somewhat different from that of the medical profession.

Perhaps the biggest concern with EBP is that healthcare professionals may not have the necessary level of skill to interpret and make use of the evidence that they find. Advances in technology and scientific research possibilities and approaches further compound this. In addition, it is anticipated that there is little time allocated for learning these skills due to the busy and stressful nature of the profession. Healthcare professionals need both the knowledge and skills to make use of the available evidence that is both timely and worthwhile.

WHAT SKILLS ARE NEEDED?

While the idea for evidence-based medicine (EBM) grew out of Cochrane's work, McMaster Medical School in Canada is credited with coining the term in 1980 to describe a particular learning approach used in the school. This approach had four steps (Peile, 2004) and these are as follows:

1. Ask an answerable question.
2. Find the appropriate evidence.
3. Critically appraise that evidence.
4. Apply the evidence to the patient, giving consideration to the individual needs, presentation and context.

In addition to this, Aas and Alexanderson (2011) suggested a 'Five A' step process (see Figure 1.3). For the purposes of this book the authors have added an additional sixth stage, that of assess; this sits at the start of the cycle whereby the clinician identifies a problem and the need for further information and action. EBP should be all about doing – tackling real problems in clinical practice.

The most important element of the cycle is the asking of the question. The question should focus on the problem, the intervention and the outcome. Herbert et al. (2012) expanded the notion of the clinical question to include:

*   effects of the intervention;
*   patients' experiences;
*   the course of the condition, or life-course (prognosis);
*   the accuracy of diagnostic tests or assessments.

Evidence-based questions are usually articulated in terms of: What is the evidence for the effectiveness of x (the intervention) for y (the outcome) in a patient with z (the problem or diagnosis)?

Taking the above together, there is a need to develop particular skills and knowledge related to:

*   the ability to identify what counts as appropriate evidence;
*   forming a question to enable you to find evidence for consideration;
*   developing a search strategy;

- finding the evidence;
- critically appraising the evidence;
- drawing on clinical expertise;
- issues concerned with patient preference;
- application to the context of care delivery;
- putting the evidence into practice.

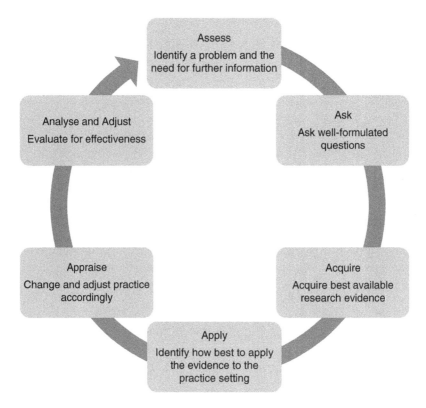

Figure 1.3   A 'Five A' plus one step approach to EBP

As part of promoting the use of EBP in clinical practice there has been a drive to develop and facilitate what have been called Communities of Practice. While the concept of communities of practice has been around for a number of years the term did not really start to take shape until the early 1990s with the work of Lave and Wenger (1991) and is largely based on the idea of learning through situated learning and the sharing of knowledge and ideas and has been defined as:

> ... a process of social learning that occurs when people who have a common interest in a subject or area collaborate over an extended period of time, sharing ideas and strategies, determine solutions, and build innovations. (Wenger, 2002: 8)

It is not so much that learners acquire structures or models to understand the world, but they participate in frameworks that have structure. The idea is centred on the notion that practitioners want to move practice forward and see the benefits of collaboration. Communities of practice will be explored in greater depth in Chapter 3: Clinical Judgement and Decision Making.

Likewise, we have seen the drive to develop Clinical Academics – health professionals who work across clinical and academic environments – to help bridge the theory–practice gap. The historical development and current opportunities for developing clinical academic careers are discussed in Chapter 11.

RESPONSIBILITY FOR EVIDENCE-BASED NURSING PRACTICE

The Canadian Nurses Association's (2009) *Position Statement on Evidence-informed Decision-making and Nursing Practice* emphasises the role that not only nurses, but other health professionals have in promoting and practising in an evidence-based way. These collaborative responsibilities go beyond the individual and extend to identifying and addressing barriers and enhancing factors within organisational structures and the healthcare system that facilitate and promote evidence-informed practice. These responsibilities are as follows:

Individual nurses

- Are positioned to provide optimal care by having acquired competencies for evidence-informed nursing practice as part of their foundational education;
- Read and critique evidence-informed literature (i.e. research articles, reports) in nursing, health sciences and related disciplines;
- Generate researchable questions and communicate them to their manager or clinical nurse leaders or associated researchers;
- Participate in or conduct research; and
- Evaluate and promote evidence-informed nursing practice.

Professional and nursing specialty associations

- Use the best available evidence as a basis for standards and guidelines;
- Lobby governments for funding to support nursing research and health information systems that include nursing care data;
- Lobby governments for healthy public policy, regulation and legislation that are evidence-informed.

Researchers

- Identify knowledge gaps and establish research priorities in conjunction with clinicians and/or other health professionals, key stakeholders and client groups;
- Generate high-quality evidence through research;
- Facilitate capacity building of new nurse researchers; and
- Engage in effective knowledge transfer, translation and exchange to communicate relevant findings of the results of research to those who require the information.

Educators and educational institutions

- Support those graduating from basic and continuing nursing education programmes to acquire competencies to provide evidence-informed nursing;
- Use and develop evidence-informed curricula by providing high-quality education in research methods, evidence collection and analysis; and
- Promote a spirit of enquiry, critical thinking, openness to change and a philosophy of lifelong learning.

Health service delivery organisations

- Reduce barriers against and enhance the factors within organisations that promote evidence-informed practice by integrating research findings and practice guidelines;
- Evaluate outcome measures through ongoing audits and formal research studies;
- Support registered nurses' involvement in research and in the transfer of research into organisational policy and practice; and
- Provide continuing education to assist nurses to maintain and increase their competence with respect to evidence-informed practice.

Governments

- Support development of health information systems that support evidence-informed nursing practice;
- Support health information institutions; and
- Provide adequate funding to support nursing research in all its phases.

Source: Canadian Nurses Association (2009) *Position Statement: Evidence-informed Decision-making and Nursing Practice*. Ottawa.

The list emphasises the prominent role that nurses, and clinicians, have to play in promoting evidence-based practice. From ensuring that their practice is up to date and based on the best evidence available, to adding their voice and weight to local and government initiatives, as well as playing an active part in and initiating research studies of their own. It also emphasises the importance of communication between groups and the need to disseminate and make use of best evidence to inform care and service provision. These topics and processes will now be explored in greater depth in the chapters that follow.

Summary

- EBP is a global phenomenon that promotes the idea of best practice, clinical effectiveness and quality care and involves an integration of evidence, clinical expertise, patient preferences and the clinical context of care delivery to inform clinical decision making.

(Continued)

- EBP focuses on critically appraising evidence to support care delivery rather than on research to discover new knowledge.
- The emergence of the expert patient has given rise to the need for health professionals to ensure they are up to date, and their care is based on the best evidence available.
- Government initiatives have promoted EBP as a way of providing both clinically effective and cost-effective healthcare.
- Various steps are associated with the EBP process – forming a question; finding evidence; critically appraising the evidence; integration of evidence into practice.
- The knowledge and skills associated with EBP are an essential component of nursing practice.

FURTHER READING

Greenhalgh, T. (2019) *How to Read a Paper: The Basics of Evidence-Based Medicine and Healthcare* (6th edn). Oxford: Wiley-Blackwell/BMJ Books.

Spruce, L. (2015) 'Back to basics: implementing evidence-based practice', *AORN Journal*, 101(1): 106–12.

USEFUL WEBLINKS

Cochrane Collaboration: promotes, supports and prepares systematic reviews, mainly in relation to effectiveness. www.cochrane.org

Joanna Briggs Institute: promotes evidence-based healthcare through systematic reviews and a range of resources aimed at promoting evidence synthesis, transfer and utilisation. https://jbi.global/

National Institute for Health and Care Excellence: provides guidance and other products to enable and support health professionals deliver evidence-based care. www.nice.org.uk

2

The Nature of Knowledge, Evidence and Ethical Approval

Ros Kane and Janet Barker

Learning Outcomes

By the end of the chapter, you will be able to:

- discuss the nature of knowledge;
- identify what is meant by 'evidence';
- understand how values-based practice complements evidence-based practice;
- demonstrate awareness of the principles of research ethics and governance.

INTRODUCTION

Knowledge is defined as: 'Facts, information, and skills acquired through experience or education; the theoretical or practical understanding of a subject' (*Oxford English Dictionary*, 2021). It is suggested that humans have a basic need for knowledge and a thirst to know how things work and why things happen. Parahoo (2014) proposed that knowledge is essential for human survival, and central to decision making about daily life and achieving change in both people and the environment in which they live. Prior to the eighteenth century much of people's understanding of the world and how it worked was based on beliefs related to superstitions and organised religions. However, the eighteenth century ushered in what we know as the era of 'Enlightenment' and the 'Age of Reason' which promoted different ways of thinking and knowing the world. The work of encyclopaedists (generally the leading philosophers of the day) and the publication of the *Encyclopedie* in the period from 1751 to

1772 together advocated scientific knowledge. This type of knowledge influenced thinking about the nature of humans and their ways of understanding the world, and from this came an opening of the debate about what knowledge is and how humans can 'know' things.

Knowledge and evidence are inextricably linked – evidence provides support to the usefulness of certain types of knowledge and knowledge gives reason and value to different forms of evidence. Therefore, as with knowledge, there are many different forms of evidence, each of which will be valued in different ways according to context.

This chapter will consider the issues surrounding the nature of knowledge, the different forms of evidence and how it is possible to identify what knowledge is needed to ensure practice is evidence based.

NATURE OF KNOWLEDGE

Knowledge is broadly categorised into two types – **propositional** and **non-propositional**. Propositional or codified knowledge is said to be public knowledge, and is often given a formal status by its inclusion in educational programmes. Non-propositional knowledge is personal knowledge linked to experience, and is described by Eraut (2000) as a 'cognitive resource' – a way of making sense of things – that someone brings to any given situation to help them think and act. It is often linked to **'tacit' knowledge**. This is knowledge that is often difficult to put into words. For instance, people may know how to ride a bike and know how they learnt to do it, but may not be able to describe critical aspects, such as how they keep their balance. In considering where knowledge comes from, Kerlinger (1999) identified three sources – **tenacity**, **authority** and **a priori**. Tenacity relates to knowledge that is believed simply because it has always been held as the truth. Authority relates to knowledge that comes from a source or person viewed as being authoritative and, therefore, must be true. A priori knowing relates to reasoning processes, where it is reasonable to consider something to be true. It is suggested that all three sources of knowledge are viewed as being objective in nature and not based on a person's subjective view of the world (see Box 2.1 for examples of these types of knowledge).

Box 2.1   Examples of three sources of knowledge

An individual with a cold knows that taking cough mixture will soothe their cough. If asked how they know this they might answer:

- 'because I know it does' - tenacity;
- 'because my mother told me it does' - authority;
- 'because it stands to reason that cough medicine will soothe a cough' - a priori.

It has been suggested that in relation to clinical decision making there are four forms of knowledge available to practitioners – superstition, folklore, craft and **science** (Justice, 2010). Superstition is similar to tenacity in that it is a belief that has no rational basis, such as the belief that bad things always happen in threes. Folklore relates more to a pattern of beliefs put forward at an earlier time, which are slow to be replaced by other, more feasible explanations for behaviours, such as the belief that the cycles of the moon affect the behaviour of people with mental health problems. Craft-based knowledge is seen most commonly as being practice-based knowledge – gained through clinical experience and drawing on personal judgement and intuition. However, there may well be a theoretical aspect, often gained during initial professional education. Science is a broad term relating to the ways of understanding the world. It is frequently thought to have a uniform definition; however, as will be discussed below, there are different views as to what can be deemed 'scientific knowledge'.

> Think about recent experiences in practice. Can you identify examples of knowledge that are based on tenacity, authority and a priori sources, and also those that appear to have their basis in superstition, folklore and craft knowledge?

Activity 2.1

PHILOSOPHICAL UNDERPINNINGS OF KNOWLEDGE AND RESEARCH

The term science comes from the Latin word *scientia*, meaning knowledge. Such knowledge has traditionally been seen as being based on observation, experiment and measurement (Mason and Mason-Whitehead, 2011). Scientific knowledge is usually generated either through **deductive** or **inductive reasoning** (Streubert and Carpenter, 2010). Deductive reasoning is said to move from the general to the particular, while inductive reasoning moves from the particular to the general. With deductive reasoning, a researcher would start with a hypothesis, which she or he would then seek to prove. A **hypothesis** is a simple statement that identifies a cause and effect relationship between two things – if I do X then Y is likely to happen. For example, in relation to considering the use of wound dressings (the general issue) a nurse might consider that one form of dressing (the particular) is more effective than another. The hypothesis might be that wound dressing A will promote more rapid wound healing than dressing B. In inductive reasoning, a nurse might start by considering somebody's experience of leg ulcers (a specific issue); she or he could then interview various people who have the condition, asking them about their experiences. Once a number of views have been collected it is possible to draw conclusions and a general theory of the experience could then be developed.

Ontology – the study of reality and how it can be understood (Ormston et al., 2018) – has evolved to encompass a range of theoretical positions on the nature of social reality and modes of apprehension: **realism** posits that there exists an external reality independent of subjective human perceptions; **materialism** (a variant of realism) proposes that reality is only perceptible through material features such as economics; while the position of **idealism** holds that reality can only be apprehended through the mind which constructs meaning or attaches it to experience.

Deductive reasoning is often associated with **positivism**, the idea that reality is ordered, regular, can be studied objectively and quantified. A basic component of positivism is **empiricism**, where it is proposed that only that which can be observed can be called fact or truth. This positivist or empirical way of looking at the world is based on a belief that 'reality' is external to and independent from humans but that humans can, by objectively observing the world around them, uncover knowledge that is true. Originally, such observation was intended to mean observation by human senses – sight, touch and so on. However, over time this has been expanded to include indirect observation through the use of specific tools designed to help a scientist observe and record phenomena. So, whereas the study of personality could be viewed as impossible because it cannot be seen, the development of a personality inventory provides a tool that the scientist can use to study it empirically. The idea of 'cause and effect' is also important in empiricism – if I do this (cause) then this (effect) will happen – so, for example, if dressing X is used (cause) the wound will heal more quickly (effect). Empiricism is often described as reductionist, which relates to the breaking down of areas of interest into small parts rather than considering the whole.

The positivist way of looking at the world developed particularly from scientific methods used in maths and physics and emphasises the need for objective and unbiased enquiry. The positivist worldview came to dominate scientific enquiry into the natural world. The more recent development of scientific enquiry into the social world (the social sciences include psychology, sociology and anthropology – these subjects explore how human beings think, behave and interact with each other and with their environment) found the positivist worldview to be limited in generating knowledge about the social world. **Interpretivism** – a different worldview – emerged from the social sciences.

Inductive reasoning is linked with interpretivism, an alternative to positivism based on the belief that humans are actively involved in constructing their understanding of the world. It is proposed that individuals constantly strive to understand what is happening in their environment and interpret action and interaction in an effort to make sense of their experiences. From this perspective, it is proposed that there is a range of views of the world and ways of understanding, depending on the interpretation people give to their experiences. Rather than adopting reductionist approaches and identifying cause and effect, interpretivism is seen as considering the whole, exploring all the subjective values and meanings that people attach to their experiences and seeking a full as possible understanding of phenomena. The interpretivist understanding is not arrived at objectively by 'pure' observation (as is the aim of the positivist worldview) but is approached inductively by exploring subjective experience. The role of the researcher using an interpretivist approach has to be acknowledged as another layer of interpretation – that is, in the process of interpreting their findings they may be influenced by their own values and experiences (Ormston et al., 2018).

As can be seen from the above, philosophical positions are adopted about the nature of the world, what can be known and how to gather this knowledge. These philosophical positions are known as **paradigms**, a term first created by Kuhn (1970). A paradigm is a set of logically connected ideas which guide the way in which research can be conducted – the methods used, the form of data collected and how those data are analysed. These design aspects of research must clearly support the uncovering of knowledge that will be perceived as having truth value. Two paradigms are generally accepted as being present in research – qualitative and quantitative – based on two different and sometimes competing ways of discovering the world. Researchers must consider carefully which paradigm or worldview best fits with the knowledge they are seeking to uncover – the design of their research must align with its purpose (LoBiondo-Wood and Haber, 2017). Qualitative research is concerned with exploring the meanings people attach to experiences and generating theories, whereas quantitative research is focused on generating data to prove or disprove theories. The paradigms are reflected in the way data are collected: put simply, qualitative data tend to be in the form of words, what people say about their experiences; quantitative data are presented in the form of numbers providing a basis for statistical analysis. Examples of how research into the same general area might look are given in Table 2.1.

Table 2.1   Examples of research questions

An investigation of anxiety in patients	
What is the nature of anxiety in patients?	Are patients who are supplied with information less anxious than those who are not?
What sorts of things provoke anxiety and what is the relationship between them?	
This is a qualitative approach ... the question is a 'what IS this?' type. Suggests an inductive approach, moving from the specific to the general.	This requires a quantitative approach. Suggests a cause and effect relationship and then tests it.

Table 2.2   Differences between quantitative and qualitative research

Quantitative	Qualitative
Scientific principles	Understanding/meaning of events
Moves from theory to data	Moves from data to theory
Identification of causal relationships between data	A close understanding of the research context
Collection of adequate amount of data	Collection of 'rich/deep' data
Application of controls to ensure validity	Seeks to address all aspects of the issues
Highly structured	Flexible structure allowing for changes in emphasis
Objectivity	Researcher as part of the process
Acceptance/rejection of hypothesis/laws	Generation of theory

Quantitative methods include randomised control trials (RCTs), experimental designs and involve statistical analysis of data. Qualitative enquiry includes phenomenology, ethnography, action research and grounded theory and generally involves interviews and observation, although some forms may incorporate aspects of statistical analysis. Table 2.2 provides a brief summary of the differences between qualitative and quantitative approaches. Issues related to the research approaches are discussed in further detail in Chapters 6 and 7.

AN EXAMPLE FROM NURSING

There is much debate as to what constitutes nursing knowledge. Knowledge plays a complex role in professions, often being seen as a defining trait. Schön (1990) suggested there is a hierarchy of knowledge in professions:

- basic science;
- applied science;
- technical skills of everyday practice.

He also suggested that professions' status is dependent on this hierarchy, that the closer a professional knowledge base is to basic science the higher the status. Nursing has tried for many years to establish a defined scientific knowledge base. Huntington and Gilmour (2001) stated that nursing has traditionally focused on empirical approaches to knowledge generation and has used these to explain the nature of nursing practice. The development of this knowledge has been influenced by other disciplines such as medicine, psychology and sociology. Although for a number of years scientific knowledge has been accepted as superior to other forms, more recently this has been challenged and there is a growing belief that other forms of knowledge are essential in the practice of nursing.

Carper (1978) was one of the first people to provide a framework through which the patterns of knowing in nursing could be considered. She identified four types of nursing knowledge – empirical, personal, aesthetic and ethical – and suggested that no one form of knowledge is superior to another; instead, each was essential to the practice of nursing. Empirical knowledge is the theoretical and research-based knowledge that is generated through systematic investigation and observation. This may also be knowledge generated by other disciplines, which can be seen as either a theory underpinning practice (such as anatomy and physiology) or a theory translated for use in nursing in a unique way (as with applied sciences such as psychology). Chinn and Kramer (2018) added the development of nursing theory to the concept of empirical knowledge, particularly in relation to interpretive research approaches such as phenomenology.

Personal knowledge relates to the individual nurse's experience of the world generally and nursing specifically. It encompasses that person's beliefs, values, perception and level of self-awareness. In many ways it resembles reflective practice, as implicit within this is the ability to know oneself and how this influences one's practice. The emotional aspects of nursing require nurses to consider how and why they respond to certain situations in certain ways to ensure the care they deliver is appropriate and compassionate. This type of knowledge is something that is seen as changing over time and having direct implications on the type and form of interactions that occur between nurses and patients.

Aesthetic knowledge is described as that knowledge which underpins the 'art' of nursing and healthcare. It can be seen as a bringing together of the manual, technical and intellectual skills aspects of nursing, particularly in nurse and patient interactions. This type of knowledge is often linked to expert practice and the ability to assist individuals in coping with health issues in a positive way.

Finally, ethical knowledge is seen as focusing on what is right, appropriate and moral; it relates to the judgements to be made in relation to nursing actions. It is also related to codes of conduct, procedural guidelines and the philosophical principles that underpin nursing.

Activity 2.2

Reflect on a recent clinical placement. Can you identify specific incidents where you used Carper's four types of knowledge?

Table 2.3 gives examples of activities associated with the different types of knowledge identified by Carper.

Intuition is an area that has been the subject of much debate, with what is termed **intuitive knowledge** being seen by many as an important aspect of clinical practice. Intuition can be defined as the 'instant understanding of knowledge without evidence of sensible thought' (Billay et al., 2007: 147) and is often considered to be a form of tacit knowledge. It is the moment when someone 'knows' that something is going to happen, or reaches a conclusion, without being aware of thinking in a rational and logical way to arrive at that point.

Table 2.3   Examples of activities associated with different types of knowledge

Knowledge	Example
Empirical	Biological sciences knowledge to understand blood pressure readings
	Psychology theory in relation to phobias to understand a patient's fear of injections/needles
Personal	'Therapeutic use of self' in understanding a person's response when given 'bad news'
	Interpersonal relationships, therapeutic relationships
Ethical	Code of conduct
	Confidentiality
Aesthetic	Communicating with a patient in a caring and appropriate way before giving an injection
	Recognising the individual needs of a person when helping them with personal hygiene

In considering the nature of intuition in professional practice, Benner (1984) suggested that a form of practice knowledge or 'expertise' exists which is part of expert practice. Here, healthcare professionals draw on all their empirical and personal knowledge to reach a conclusion, without being aware of processing the information (see Box 2.2 for an example). Benner differentiates between practical and theoretical knowledge, suggesting that the former relates to 'knowing how' and is related to skills and the latter to 'knowing that', which is concerned with the generation of theory and scientific knowledge. However, she also suggested that in nursing, as expertise develops, a form of practice knowledge is apparent that 'side steps' the logical reasoning processes associated with science. Extending the knowing how through practice experience can lead to knowledge that appears to be available to the person without the aid of analytical process, but which nevertheless is valid.

> ### Box 2.2   Example of expert knowledge (Benner, 1984: 32)
>
> An extract from an interview with a nurse who worked in the psychiatric setting for 15 years:
>
> When I say to a doctor 'this patient is psychotic', I don't always know how to legitimise that statement. But I am never wrong. Because I know psychosis from inside out. And I feel that, and I know it, and I trust it. I don't care if nothing else is happening, I still really know that. It's like the feeling another nurse described in the small group interview today, when she said about the patient 'she just isn't right'.

Other forms of knowing have been added to Carper's original work. For example, Mullhall (1993) put forward the idea of 'unknowing', proposing that nurses needed to make deliberate attempts to be open to new ideas and ways of thinking; seeing this as a step in building knowledge and a deeper understanding of individual practice experiences. Socio-political knowledge was included by White (1995). Here, political awareness, cultural diversity and public health agendas are essential aspects of knowing, enabling nursing to see its practice in a broader arena. Chinn and Kramer (2018) proposed 'emancipatory knowledge', that is, an awareness of social inequalities and their implication for health, including a political awareness, the need for social change and methods to bring this about.

WHAT CONSTITUTES EVIDENCE?

The dictionary definition of evidence is 'The available body of facts or information indicating whether a belief or proposition is true or valid' (*Oxford English Dictionary*, 2021). Pearson (2005) proposed in healthcare that it is 'data or information used to decide whether or not a claim or view should be trusted'. What exactly constitutes evidence in EBP is still hotly debated. Thomas (2004) suggested that evidence is information that is seen as relevant to how to provide care and beliefs about health and illness. Various hierarchies of evidence have been generated which clearly place quantitative findings from systematic reviews of RCTs at the top of the hierarchy; often qualitative research findings are not included within these hierarchies at all (see Chapter 4 for a more detailed discussion of evidence hierarchies). This preference for one form of evidence over another perhaps comes from the Cochrane Collaboration, which focused on the effectiveness of interventions for which RCTs are ideally suited and also on the dominance of the positivist paradigm in terms of research approaches. However, there is a growing body of literature that hotly contests the placing of RCT methods at the top of the hierarchy. Scott and McSherry (2008) suggested that RCTs are not always the most pertinent approach to certain aspects of nursing care. As discussed above, different ways of exploring the natural and the social worlds have developed and the practice of nursing encompasses both natural and social sciences.

Porter and O'Halloran (2012) assert that RCTs do not provide the best evidence for the complex systems in which healthcare is delivered. Different types of research questions require different forms of study. Therefore, the most appropriate form of evidence is that which relates to the question being asked – 'horses for courses' as Petticrew and Roberts (2003) put it.

Nursing has long recognised that its practice is based on multiple ways of knowing, and much of nursing activity does not fit easily with an RCT approach. The advocating of one type of evidence as superior to another is not helpful in providing evidence on which to base practice in a profession as multifaceted and complex as nursing. It is suggested that perhaps it is more appropriate to acknowledge the possibility of multiple hierarchies, depending on the object or issue under consideration. Nairn (2012: 14) proposed 'there is one world, but multiple ways of examining that world'.

The Joanna Briggs Institute (JBI) supports the idea of there being a range of issues that need to be considered in healthcare, and that different forms of evidence are needed. It is suggested that evidence generally falls into four areas:

1. Evidence of feasibility – whether something is practical/practicable physically, culturally or financially. In this situation one type of treatment might be the most effective, but financially unaffordable. For example, the cost of certain drugs means they are not used in certain healthcare systems. Types of evidence to support this would probably be economic and policy research.
2. Evidence of appropriateness – whether a particular intervention fits with the context in which it is to be given. For example, blood transfusion within certain religious groups might not be an appropriate form of treatment. Research considering ethical and philosophical issues would be of use here.
3. Evidence of meaningfulness – how interventions/activities are experienced by individuals. For example, the patients' experiences of or beliefs about fertility treatment might influence how services are organised. Interpretive research in the form of phenomenology, ethnology or grounded theory would be of interest in this area.
4. Evidence of effectiveness – whether one treatment is better than another or the usual intervention. RCTs and cohort studies would be of use here.

Rycroft-Malone et al. (2004) suggested four types of evidence on which nurses can base their practice:

1. Research.
2. Clinical experience.
3. Service user/carer perspectives.
4. Local context.

They went on to identify that the challenge is in knowing how to integrate these four types of evidence in a robust and patient-centred way.

Ensuring the robustness of evidence related to clinical experience requires the gathering and documenting of this experience in a systematic manner, allowing for individual and group reflection and cross-checking. Portfolios and clinical supervision are methods which can enhance the validity of this type of evidence and these are explored further in Chapter 11.

A crucial skill for nurses to develop is the ability to scrutinise and critically evaluate the quality of evidence. Chapter 5 introduces a number of research tools which help to develop these skills and can be of use in practice.

THE ROLE OF VALUES

Recent scrutiny of the NHS in the UK has led to a recognition of the need to reflect on current culture and practice and the revisiting of the values which underpin practice (McGonagle et al., 2015). In England, the Department of Health and Social Care has set out a commitment to values in the NHS Constitution (DHSC, 2021). Central to this is the understanding that patients are at the core of decision making, not simply passive recipients of care or treatment.

Values-based practice (VBP) is an approach to healthcare delivery that seeks to complement evidence-based practice (EBP) (Fulford, 2008). It is the utilisation of skills to promote balanced decision making in patient care, while also accounting for the complex web of differing value perspectives which lie behind the decision-making process. Much has been written about the place of VBP in the delivery of care (Fulford et al., 2012). It is predicated on the belief that different perspectives need to be respected, especially when dealing with challenging topics. The respect for alternative points of view (including the patient's) is seen as an opportunity to open dialogue and positively challenge and reflect on personal, societal and organisational values, attitudes and behaviours.

The drive to EBP is a highly desirable aspect of modern health services. However, it has been argued that it has minimised the role that values have in care delivery (Woodbridge and Fulford, 2004). It is rare that the evidence base for practice comes 'value free' (Fulford and Stanghellini, 2008). It is argued, therefore, that the drive for clinical quality through EBP must be delivered with a drive for values too (McGonagle et al., 2015).

Incorporating sources of evidence from patients, the public and carers into the delivery of care has a long tradition within nursing and underpins the ethos of holistic care. Their inclusion in research is also now recognised as essential (see www.learningforinvolvement. org.uk/ for guidance on how to involve the public in health and social care research). However, this source of evidence has its own inherent complexities and can be challenging. When research findings promoting the view that a specific form of intervention is most appropriate (for example, the use of a particular medication in managing mental health problems) are at odds with the service user's experience (the medication has specific side effects that make the person unwilling to take it), the clinical expertise of the nurse is essential in identifying the most appropriate course of action.

Institutional cultures, social and professional networks, evaluations such as 360-degree feedback and local/national policies are some of the forms of evidence found in the local setting (Rycroft-Malone et al., 2004). Other relevant local evidence includes audits and individual patient preferences and service evaluations.

There are also some 'ready-made' forms of evidence available, where best evidence has been collected and summarised for use by healthcare professionals. Clinical Knowledge Summaries, produced by the National Institute for Health and Care Excellence (NICE) are an example of this type of resource. This is an online collection of concise summaries of available evidence, providing recommendations on how to manage commonly encountered clinical situations in care settings (see https://cks.nice.org.uk/). It is also possible to sign up for alerts to specific areas of evidence as it is published (see https://evidence.nihr.ac.uk/alerts/).

A further initiative is the publication of BITEs (Brokering Innovation Through Evidence), which have been developed by the Applied Research Collaboration (ARC) as a means of conveying the 'need to know' information about a piece of research to busy clinicians and health and social care staff (see https://arc-em.nihr.ac.uk/resources?resource%5B%5D=39).

A relatively new initiative in EBP is that of **care bundles**. Here, elements of best practice evidence (usually between three and five) are grouped together in relation to a particular condition, treatment and/or procedure. These elements are ones that are generally used in practice but not necessarily applied in the same way or combination to all appropriate patients. Care bundles 'tie' together these elements into a unit that is delivered to every patient in the same way. Dawson and Endacott (2011) identified that combining elements in this way has a more positive impact on treatment outcomes than any one single element. They suggested that care bundles appear to be more effective than clinical guidelines in improving possible outcomes, as the former are seen as mandatory while the latter are often viewed as purely advisory.

Care bundles were originally developed in 2002 at the Johns Hopkins University in the USA in relation to critical care environments. It was found that using four interventions with patients on ventilators significantly reduced length of stay and number of ventilator days. Care bundles have now also been developed in a number of other areas, such as infection control, and are advocated by the Department of Health and Social Care as a tool for high impact change. However, the then Institute for Healthcare Improvement (2012) warned against an ad hoc approach to bringing elements of care together, stressing that the strength of the bundles lies in the underpinning science, the way it is delivered and consistency in its application.

QUESTIONS

Having identified what counts as good evidence, the next task is to find the evidence. This requires the formulating of a relevant question (see Chapter 4), often considered the backbone of EBP. Ideas in relation to questions about practice can come from a range of situations, reflection on practice issues, audit outcomes and discussions between nurses, patients and/or other health professionals. Often, such questions are broad and unfocused, but if appropriate answers are to be found, then there is a need to develop specific, focused research questions.

You are currently working in a residential care setting. Mary, a 66-year-old patient in your care, has fallen and fractured her femur. In discussion with the rest of the care staff it is identified that there have been a number of falls over the year that have resulted in fractured femurs. Someone remembers

(Continued)

Activity 2.3

reading about 'hip protectors' as a method of reducing injuries. You have been asked to look for some evidence to help make decisions as to how to address the issues. Where would you start? Reflect on this scenario and start to think about the types of unanswered research questions that might arise.

An obvious starting place might be to go online and Google the words 'fractured femur', but this is likely to produce thousands of hits or nothing at all. There is a need to focus the search to ensure that the relevant information is obtained while vital pieces of information are not missed. Chapter 4 goes into more detail, with worked examples of how to formulate specific research questions. Apply this scenario using the frameworks introduced.

Stillwell et al. (2010) identified two forms of questions that practitioners might ask – **background** and **foreground**. Background questions are generally broad and have two parts:

1. The question's stem – who, what, where, when, how, why?
2. The area of clinical interest.

A background question might look something like 'What is the best way of treating depression?' There is a need to ask background questions, particularly for students and those new to an area of practice, in order to gain the knowledge and expertise needed in relation to a specific area. The problem with background questions is their broadness, which makes it difficult to find specific information, and searching for information is often done in a haphazard way – indeed, it is easy to end up looking in the wrong place.

Foreground questions ask about specific issues and are looking for particular knowledge. A foreground question might be something like 'Which is more effective in treating depression – cognitive behavioural therapy or medication?'

It is essential that a foreground question is formulated containing all the key elements for consideration, before searching the literature in relation to a particular issue. The question will be central to ensuring that the search is not too broad, which in turn may result in retrieving an overwhelming amount of literature, or too narrow in scope, resulting in key items being missed. There are a number of formats that can be used to help to create a search question and these are discussed in more detail in Chapter 4.

Activity 2.4

Think about a recent clinical experience and identify a patient whose care you were closely involved with. Focusing on one clinical intervention you undertook in relation to this person (giving an injection, attending to hygiene needs, involvement of patients in recreational/therapeutic activities), write a reflective account identifying:

1. What knowledge you were using during the intervention/activity, considering what areas of knowledge you felt most comfortable with and those that you need to develop further.
2. What evidence you used to direct how you organised your intervention/activity.
3. The questions you would ask if you wanted to find further evidence to support your practice in this area.

RESEARCH GOVERNANCE AND ETHICS

Anyone undertaking research needs to be aware of the principles of research ethics and governance. This is discussed in more detail in Chapter 5. Essentially, in the UK, the Health Research Authority (HRA) and the Devolved UK Administrations have developed a UK Policy Framework for Health and Social Care Research which sets out the high-level principles of good practice in the management and conduct of health and social care research in the UK, as well as the responsibilities that underpin high-quality ethical research (HRA, 2020). A core standard for healthcare organisations is that they have systems to ensure the principles and requirements of this research governance framework are consistently applied. The HRA is a central resource to guide aspects of healthcare research and also provides guidance to ensure that studies comply with the General Data Protection Regulations (2018) (see www.hra.nhs.uk/planning-and-improving-research/policies-standards-legislation/data-protection-and-information-governance/gdpr-guidance/). Useful templates which can be used for the development of ethics applications are also freely available. As such, in the UK, all NHS organisations will have a Research Governance Department, which is an essential port of call for any employees looking to undertake research. Research Governance Departments will offer advice on the process for applying for ethical approval both locally and, where needed, nationally through the NHS integrated research application system (see www.myresearchproject.org.uk/). Crucially, Research Governance staff will help individuals to ascertain the level of approvals required before undertaking any data collection. This varies by the nature of the project being undertaken. For example, health professionals are increasingly undertaking service improvement projects or service evaluations, which may not need to be submitted to the HRA, but rather can be approved by local Research Governance Departments. A key is to determine whether a proposed project is classified as Research, Service Evaluation/Improvement or Clinical Audit. One of the first steps in deciding which approvals are needed is therefore to determine whether it is classed as research, and therefore whether it should be managed as such. The responsibility for determining whether a project is classed as research lies with the managing organisation. To assist in this the HRA has published an interactive decision tool (www.hra-decisiontools.org.uk/research/). The tool in turn is based on the defining research table which can be found here: www.hra-decisiontools.org.uk/research/docs/DefiningResearchTable_Oct2017-1.pdf

Researchers have a responsibility to explain and justify their activities – to convey to others that their area of enquiry is both important and necessary and how they decide upon the focus of their research (Moule et al., 2016). Systems of governance and ethical approval are essential to this process, particularly in providing scrutiny over any potential for harm to those who take part in research.

Summary

- Knowledge is broadly categorised into two types – propositional (formal) and non-propositional (personal) – and comes from three sources – tenacity, authority and a priori. Clinical knowledge can be seen as based on superstition, folklore, craft or science.
- Science is a body of knowledge organised in a systematic way based on observation, experiment and measurement.
- Evidence is information or data that supports or refutes beliefs in relation to a particular area of interest.
- Evidence on which to base clinical practice is best drawn from a variety of credible sources reflecting the multifaceted and complex needs of delivering care. There are four types of evidence on which nurses and other healthcare professionals can base their practice – research, clinical experience, service user/carer perspectives and local context.
- There are 'ready-made' forms of evidence available, where best evidence has been collected and summarised, such as clinical guidelines and summaries.
- All clinical staff involved in research must familiarise themselves with local and national principles of research governance and ethics application processes.

FURTHER READING

Carper, B. (1978) 'Fundamental patterns of knowing in nursing', *Advances in Nursing Science*, 1: 13–23.

Health Research Authority (HRA) (2020) *UK Policy Framework for Health and Social Care Research*. Health Research Authority. www.hra.nhs.uk/planning-and-improving-research/policies-standards-legislation/uk-policy-framework-health-social-care-research/

USEFUL WEBLINKS

The Collaborating Centre for Values-Based Practise in Health and Social Care was set up to support the development of values-based practice through shared learning. Based at St Catherine's College in Oxford the Centre brings together a wide range of individuals and organisations working on different aspects of values-based practice around the world. https://valuesbasedpractice.org/

Clinical Knowledge Summaries: provides concise summaries of evidence related to common primary care issues and gives recommendations for practice. http://cks.nice.org.uk/#?char=A

Good Clinical Practice Training: Good Clinical Practice (GCP) is the international ethical, scientific and practical standard to which all clinical research is conducted and training by the National Institute for Health Research in England can be accessed here: www.nihr.ac.uk/health-and-care-professionals/learning-and-support/good-clinical-practice.htm

The Health Research Authority (HRA): a body of the Department of Health in the UK, set up to protect and promote the interests of patients and the public in health and social care research. It has published or made available a number of key resources about good research practice. www.hra.nhs.uk/

The Joanna Briggs Institute (JBI) is an international research organisation based in the Faculty of Health and Medical Sciences at the University of Adelaide, South Australia. It develops and delivers unique evidence-based information, software, education and training designed to improve healthcare practice and health outcomes. https://jbi.global/

Learning for Involvement is funded by the National Institute for Health Research in England and dedicated to learning and development for public involvement in health and social care research and provides a wide range of free resources. www.learningforinvolvement.org.uk/

NHS Evidence: enables users to simultaneously search 150 data sources for resources such as clinical summaries, guidelines, research literature, the British National Formulary. www.evidence.nhs.uk

Trip Database: a search engine that identifies high-quality evidence for use in clinical practice. www.tripdatabase.com

The Institute for Healthcare Improvement (IHI) is a long-established global organisation which uses improvement science to advance and sustain better outcomes in health and healthcare across the world. www.ihi.org

3

Clinical Judgement and Decision Making

Paul Linsley

Learning Outcomes

By the end of the chapter, you will be able to:

- discuss the nature of clinical judgement and decision making;
- recognise the processes involved in clinical judgement and decision making;
- identify and use appropriate decision-making frameworks.

INTRODUCTION

Health and social care communities continually produce large amounts of research leading to revised methods of treatment and care for patients; however, this research does not always translate into clinical practice or changes to service delivery (Kristensen et al., 2016). Associated with this problem of providing for change is the increasing concern that is being felt for effectiveness and efficiency in care and treatment planning and decision making. In order to bridge what has been termed this 'theory–practice gap' (Monaghan, 2015), any changes in thinking brought about by new research must eventually be made actionable and usable, and adapted to local practice, in order to produce the desired outcome over time. This often requires nurses and other healthcare professionals to take a lead in putting the evidence into practice and making the required changes. These demands entail an increasing degree of professionalism, as well as a framework within which decisions can be reached. EBP provides such a framework for decision making and this is one of the reasons why it is heavily promoted in the literature and by professional bodies the world over. This chapter will look at clinical judgement and decision making as part of EBP.

Evidence-based decision making has been described as 'a process for making decisions about a programme, practice, or policy that is grounded in the best available evidence and informed by experiential evidence from the field and relevant contextual evidence' (Jennings and Hall, 2011: 245). This approach stands in contrast to opinion-based decisions and the untested views and ideas of individuals or groups, 'often inspired by ideological standpoints, prejudices, or speculative conjecture' (Davies, 2004: 3). It has been suggested that evidence-based practice is mediated and actioned by an interplay between individuals, new knowledge and the actual context in which the evidence is to be operationalised and utilised as part of daily practice (Sandstrom et al., 2015). Furthermore, decisions concerned with care and treatment planning call for a deep understanding and concern for people and necessitate balancing the social and task requirements of the profession and organisation to which the nurse belongs.

Prior to the advent of EBP most health professionals based clinical decision making on 'their vast educational knowledge coupled with intelligent guesswork, hunches and experience' (Pape, 2003: 155). Reliance on such approaches is no longer seen as appropriate due to a number of factors, particularly over-confidence (Lehane et al., 2018). Nursing not only involves knowing the how and why of delivering a certain type of care but also the ability to give sound rationales and justifications for clinical judgements and decisions taken. Melnyk and Fineout-Overholt (2018) have stated that it is useful to think of EBP as requiring clinicians to be involved in two essential activities regarding decision making – critically appraising evidence (discussed in Chapter 5) and using clinical judgement to consider how applicable the evidence is to their own area of practice.

In its simplest terms, decision making involves determining precise and concrete goals or objectives, and then selecting, from alternatives, a course of action that is most likely to lead to a successful outcome. However, decision making is not a straightforward activity. Clinical decisions are often characterised by situations of uncertainty where not all the information needed to make them is, or can be, known.

The increasing complexity of the care needs of individuals, care interventions and care delivery settings requires finely honed clinical judgement skills to ensure clinical decision making is of the highest standard. Lamb and Sevdalis (2011) have identified that clinical judgement and decision-making skills take practitioners beyond purely technical or knowledge-based skills, proposing these to be 'key non-technical' skills essential for the safe delivery of care. Decisions of this kind also call for a great amount of creative and imaginative thinking and cover a wide range of activities. Two approaches would seem to dominate practitioner clinical decision making. The first is the reliance on clinical expertise and intuition gained through experience and doing the job. The second is the use of actuarial decision aids. This is the use of a formula based on empirically established relations of cause and effect. It should be noted that such a formula doesn't exclude clinical judgements if those judgements have value.

WHAT IS CLINICAL JUDGEMENT?

As identified above, clinical judgement is an essential skill for all health professionals and one that separates them from undertaking a purely technical role. Various terms are used in relation to this activity (clinical reasoning, problem solving and critical thinking) but all are related to the ability to consider the various issues at hand, make a judgement in relation to the impact of the various elements and come up with a decision as to what is the appropriate action to take. A useful definition of clinical judgement is that proposed by Tanner (2006: 204), who defined it as the 'interpretation or conclusion about a patient's needs, concerns, or health problems, and/or the decision to take action (or not), use or modify standard approaches, or improvise new ones as deemed appropriate by the patient's responses'. Levett-Jones et al. (2010) suggested there are five 'rights' in relation to this concept – right cues, right patient, right action, right time for the right reason. The important thing is to make structured decisions based on sound clinical judgement. Decisions will have implications for patient outcomes and as such must deserve serious consideration.

The number and type of decisions that nurses and other healthcare professionals face are determined to some extent by their understanding and perception of their work, operational autonomy, and the degree to which they see themselves as active and influential decision makers. Thompson (2003) identified that nurses make clinical decisions in six key areas:

1. Intervention/effectiveness: choosing between intervention X and intervention Y.
2. Targeting: these decisions relate to 'choosing which patient will benefit the most from this intervention'.
3. Timing: these commonly take the form of choosing the best time to deploy particular interventions.
4. Communication: these decisions focus on choices relating to ways of delivering and receiving information to and from patients, families and colleagues. Most often these decisions relate to the communication of risks and benefits of different interventions or prognostic categories.
5. Service organisation, delivery and management: decisions concerning the configuration or processes of service delivery.
6. Experimental, understanding or hermeneutic: these decisions relate to the interpretation of cues in the process of care. The choices involved might include deciding on the ways in which a patient may be experiencing a particular situation, and are intuitive to some extent.

However, no decision should ever be made without an accompanying judgement as to the appropriateness of that decision (Van Graan and Williams, 2017).

Activity 3.1

Before reading any more of this chapter, answer the following questions: Is there a particular journal that you read on a regular basis or subscribe to? How do you put what you have read into practice? How does this affect the way in which you make clinical decisions?

In any two clinical situations the context and individual nurse's experience/knowledge will impact on the judgements and decisions made. All clinical judgements have ethical considerations, with the health professional weighing up the potential benefits and risks involved in any decision made. Frequently there are a number of options available, each of which carries its own risks and benefits. This adds another dimension to the decision-making process, and often it is the patient's preferences that indicate which is the best choice of action. However, to rely solely on this 'knowledge' for the purposes of decision making can lead to complacency (and mistakes) and fails to recognise others as individuals.

The reasoning processes used in clinical judgement tend to be described as involving either analytical or intuitive activities (Muntean, 2012). The former involves the breaking down of a problem into its constituent parts, considering these, and weighing up the alternative approaches available in solving the problem. Usually, this involves the processing of scientific data. Intuitive processes are seen as drawing on inherent knowledge, skills and experiences to find the answer to the problem. These two options are often seen as the opposite poles of a continuum. However, the idea of a 'cognitive continuum' is possibly more helpful in understanding the processes involved as these two activities are not 'mutually exclusive' (Standing, 2017). The more complex, familiar or urgent the issue the more likely you are to rely on intuition. Any combination of these three elements will result in the use of differing levels of analysis and/or intuition.

Identify and record:

- a situation where you have made a clinical decision on an emotional or biased basis;
- your actions as a result of this;
- the resulting care that followed.

Activity 3.2

Standing (2017) provided a cognitive continuum of clinical judgement in nursing based on identifying nine cognitive modes used by nurses in practice (see Table 3.1). No one mode is seen as more important than another; these simply reflected the types of knowledge drawn on in the clinical judgement and decision-making processes of nurses and the sort of activities nurses are likely to engage in. The intuitive mode is seen most frequently in face-to-face encounters with patients, whereas the experimental research mode is related to establishing effectiveness of intervention and is more distant from day-to-day care activities.

Table 3.1 Cognitive modes of nursing practice

Judgement process	Description
Intuitive	Drawing on tacit knowledge and arriving at a judgement without being aware of the process by which it was reached. Usually occurs in face-to-face care delivery situations.
Reflective	Incorporates both reflection in and on care delivery actions.
Patient and peer assisted	Encompasses seeking patient preferences and/or the expertise of other healthcare professionals.
System assisted	Involves the use of guidelines, problem-solving frameworks and decision aids.

(Continued)

Table 3.1   (Continued)

Judgement process	Description
Critical review of evidence (experience and research)	Identification of relevant information and application of this to the current situation.
Action research and audit	Gathering information through implementing and evaluating changes to care delivery systems.
Qualitative research	Seeking to understand the patient's experience and inform future practice by undertaking qualitative research.
Survey research	Answering questions related to future care delivery by collecting data via surveys.
Experimental research	Testing the effectiveness of intervention through the use of experimental research designs such as RCTs.

It has been proposed that an over-reliance on intuition may give rise to problems associated with bias – an under- or over-estimation of the importance of certain factors or information. Bias in the form of stereotyping, prejudice or selective memory can influence how you perceive and respond to information and individual patients. Equally, basing judgements and decisions purely on personal experience and knowledge results in important research evidence being ignored or undervalued. Reliance on past experience while playing an important part in clinical decision making can also impede clinical judgement if not challenged in any way (Kozlowski et al., 2017). Good decisions can only be evaluated against future events, while experience belongs to the past. This does not mean to say that experience is to be discounted, only that it is but one guide to action. It is, therefore, essential that nurses and healthcare professionals can defend judgements and justify how they reached these and the decisions made.

WHAT IS CLINICAL DECISION MAKING?

Standing (2017) proposed that clinical judgement and clinical decision making are closely linked but separate concepts. The former is about an evaluation of a situation, and the latter is concerned with whether or not to take action and what type of action to take if necessary. For example, one might consider that a particular patient's diet is poor (judgement) and choose to provide them with an education package related to healthy eating (decision). Benner et al. (1996: 2) suggested that clinical judgement relates to 'the ways in which nurses come to understand the problems, issues, or concerns of clients/patients, to attend to salient information and to respond in concerned and involved ways'. In this way decision making is seen as an interaction between three things – the patient's preferences; the evidence available on which to base practice; and the clinical judgement of the nurse involved based on personal experience and knowledge. These three components come together to produce a clinical decision as to what action should be taken – see Figure 3.1.

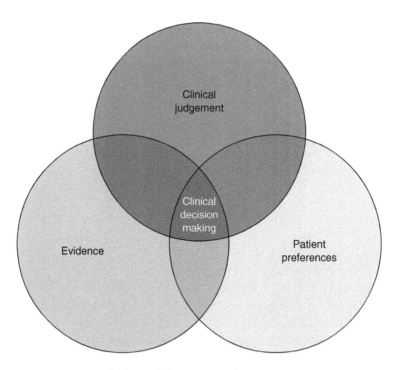

Figure 3.1   Components of clinical decision making

The core skills relating to good decision making have been identified as:

- Pattern recognition: learning from experience.
- Critical thinking: removing emotion from our reasoning, being 'sceptical', questioning and not taking things at face value, examining assumptions, being open-minded and receptive to change, and lastly being able to evaluate the evidence.
- Communication skills: active listening – listening to the patient, what they say, and what they don't say; and adopting and pursuing a patient-centred approach – the ability to provide information in a comprehensive way to allow patients, their carers and family to be involved in the decision-making process.
- Teamwork: using the gathered evidence to enlist help, support and advice from colleagues and the wider multidisciplinary team.
- Sharing: learning and getting feedback from colleagues on your decision making.
- Reflection: using feedback from others and the outcomes of the decisions to reflect on the decisions that were taken in order to enhance practice delivery in the future.

(Adapted from NHS Scottish Executive, 2006)

A number of factors would seem to influence evidence-based decision making, the more prominent of these being:

- Knowing the evidence: there are a wide variety of online journals, books and reference materials you can utilise to research the evidence base.
- Knowing yourself: being aware of your behaviour, competencies, attitudes, emotions and values and not just your own but also those of your patients/clients and colleagues.

It is also important to know your limitations – being aware of when to seek help, advice and support. Remember – you are part of a team.

- Knowing the Patient and Person: knowing the patient's preferences, their experiences of illness and their current situation or care needs and what is normal for that patient in terms of observation, mobility and level of function. It is important to consider feedback from decision-making tools that you can use to capture patient information and analyse results. Also, adhering to the rights of the patients.
- Knowing the environment: awareness and recognition of the approach to decision making and the wider team dynamics within your organisation.

(Adapted from NHS Education for Scotland, 2021)

Activity 3.3

Consider the last clinical decision you made. How did you arrive at the decision? Were you aware of analysing the various aspects of the issue or was it reached more intuitively? Did you make the judgement and decision objectively, using all the data and evidence to hand? Did your personal attitudes or biases have a part to play in the decision? Did you involve the patient in the decision-making process – from the initial information gathering to agreeing a course of action? Examine your own decision-making patterns.

The nursing process of assess, plan, implement and evaluate requires quality decision making. For example, during the assessment phase of the cycle, increased knowledge on the part of the nurse leads to greater clinical currency and judgement. The more experienced nurse knows what to look for based upon clinical knowledge and personal experience and can use this information alongside the available evidence, policy and procedure to inform the care that they give. Evaluation ensures that decisions are reviewed, and lessons are learnt. A good decision from an evidence-based perspective is one that successfully integrates four elements:

1. Professional expertise ('know–how' knowledge).
2. The available resources.
3. The patient's (informed) values.
4. The research knowledge ('know–what' knowledge).

Poor decision making in nursing usually happens when nurses use the wrong type of information to inform their decisions or place too much emphasis on a particular form of information (Dowding and Thompson, 2004). Therefore, it is crucial to ensure that when making decisions the appropriate sources of information are accessed. There are many different types of clinical decisions which nurses are called upon to make. Thompson et al. (2004) identified 11 different forms of decisions made in everyday practice (see Table 3.2).

Table 3.2 Forms of decisions made in practice

Intervention	Targeting	Timing	Prevention
Referral	Communication	Assessment	Diagnosis
Information	Experience	Service delivery	

Reflect on one recent day in clinical practice and consider if, when and how you were involved in the 11 types of decisions identified in Table 3.2. Identify how these decisions were made and whether you felt you had the appropriate evidence on which to base those decisions.

Activity 3.4

There are various conceptual models available to explain the factors involved in making a clinical decision. Tanner (2006) proposed that it is a four-stage process involving noticing, interpreting, responding and reflecting. Lasater (2007) identifies that each of these stages has specific components:

1. Noticing: observing, noticing change and collecting information.
2. Interpreting: making sense of the information and prioritising.
3. Responding: planning intervention, using clear communication and appropriate skills.
4. Reflecting: evaluating the incident and looking for ways to improve performance.

Standing (2017) suggested that clinical decision-making skills have 12 facets (see Table 3.3).

Table 3.3 Clinical decision-making skills

Collaboration	Experience and intuition	Confidence	Prevention
Systematic	Prioritising	Observation	Diagnosis
Standardisation	Reflectivity	Ethical sensitivity	Accountability

Identify one patient whose care you were recently involved with. Consider each of Standing's decision-making skills and identify whether or not you used these in making care delivery decisions.

Activity 3.5

In making a clinical decision, it is proposed that a nurse's judgement is helped if the most up-to-date evidence is available and the needs of the service user are clearly identified. However, simply providing nurses with appropriate evidence will not in itself enhance the decision-making processes. If decision making is to be effective, then health professionals need to be aware of such changes and factor them into any decisions to be made. Therefore, it is necessary to consider the implications of a decision over time – what Melnyk and Fineout-Overholt (2018) describe as 'clinical forethought'. This has four components – future think, forethought about specific populations, anticipation of risks and the unexpected (see Table 3.4 for an overview). Issues that may have an impact on, and implications for, care delivery should be identified and considered. Clinical judgement is used in managing these uncertainties and arriving at a decision as to how to proceed – many see this as the 'art' of nursing – and is central to clinical expertise.

Table 3.4   Clinical forethought

Type	Description
Future think	Considering the immediate future and anticipating issues that might arise
	Identifying immediate resources needed
	Considering future responses
	Evaluating judgement and making adjustments as necessary
Specific patients	Considering general trends in patient experiences and responses to intervention
	Identifying local resources available to deal with potential issues
Risks	Anticipating particular issues that may impact on a specific individual – such as anxiety, distress
The unexpected	Expecting the unexpected
	Anticipating the need to respond to new situations and resources – yours and organisational – if difficulties arise

Activity 3.6

Imagine you are about to administer a new form of medication to a patient for the first time. What 'clinical forethought' issues can you identify?

As identified above, nurses' personal knowledge and experience have the greatest impact on these decision-making activities, moulding how the nurse interprets the situation and deals with the uncertainties.

Nursing expertise is defined by Higgs and Titchen (2001: 274) as the 'professional artistry and practice wisdom inherent in professional practice'. Clinical expertise is viewed by Manley et al. (2005) as having a number of components (see Box 3.1). The development of these aspects of clinical expertise are said to be linked to 'enabling factors' – the ability to reflect; to organise practice giving consideration to overarching influences; to work autonomously; to develop good interpersonal relationships; and to promote respect.

Box 3.1 Nursing expertise

1. Holistic practice knowledge – integrating various forms of knowledge, academic and experiential, into their delivery of care.
2. Knowing the patient – respecting the patient's views/perspectives, encouraging patient decision making and promoting independence.
3. Moral agency promoting respect, dignity and self-efficacy in others whilst maintaining one's own professional integrity.
4. Saliency – observing and picking up on cues from patients, recognising the needs of patients and others.
5. Skilled know-how – problem solving, responding to the changing environment of care and adapting to needs as appropriate.
6. Change catalyst – promoting appropriate change.
7. Risk taker – weighing the risks and taking appropriate decisions, to achieve best patient outcomes.

APPROACHES TO DECISION MAKING

There are a number of frameworks that can be used to help with decision making.

Facione and Gittens (2013: 47) offered a five-step approach to effective thinking and problem solving known as IDEAS:

I = IDENTIFY the Problem and Set Priorities (Step 1)

D = DEEPEN Understanding and Gather Relevant Information (Step 2)

E = ENUMERATE Options and Anticipate Consequences (Step 3)

A = ASSESS the Situation and Make a Preliminary Decision (Step 4)

S = SCRUTINISE the Process and Self-Correct as Needed (Step 5)

Consider an area of concern in your area of practice. Using Facione and Gittens's framework, identify how best to address the issues of concern.

Activity 3.7

Hoffman et al. (2010) proposed a clinical reasoning cycle, based on research concerning expert nurses' thought and decision-making processes. It was suggested that this cycle can be used to promote the development of practice-specific knowledge and clinical reasoning skills in students and novice practitioners. There are eight steps in the cycle:

1. Describe the patient and the context of their care situation.
2. Consider all the information currently available (notes, charts, history) and gather any further information needed. Apply the theoretical knowledge you already have to the patient's illness/presentation and the situation.
3. Review all the data you have to get a full picture of the patient and their context. Identify what is and is not relevant, and any patterns and relationships between the various pieces of information. Compare the current situation to your past experiences and suggest possible outcomes.
4. Evaluate the information to clarify the nature of the problem to be addressed.
5. Set your goals and time frame within which these will be achieved.
6. Implement your plan of action.
7. Evaluate outcomes.
8. Reflect on the experience and identify learning needs.

Activity 3.8

Using Hoffman et al.'s framework above reflect on how you went about generating an understanding and knowledge of a patient that you looked after and how this informed the treatment and care you gave.

Carroll and Johnson (1990) suggested an alternative seven-stage model of decision making, which does not follow a linear pattern but can be repeated or returned to as necessary:

1. Recognition of the situation.
2. Formulation of explanation.
3. Alternative generation of other explanations.
4. Information search to clarify choices and available evidence.
5. Judgement or choice.
6. Action.
7. Feedback.

Activity 3.9

Think about the above three frameworks and decide which one reflects your decision-making process in clinical practice. Also see Appendix 1.

EBP calls for a more analytical approach to making clinical decisions, and it is anticipated there will be a conscious weighing up of the options and consideration of the various issues. The McMaster's EBM group caution against the use of clinical experience and intuition in the absence of evidence based on systematic observation in making clinical judgements (Eraut, 2000). However, it should not be underestimated how much interpretation may be needed in deciding how evidence should be used – EBP cannot always provide concrete evidence on which to base practice. A possible model for this process is given in Figure 3.2.

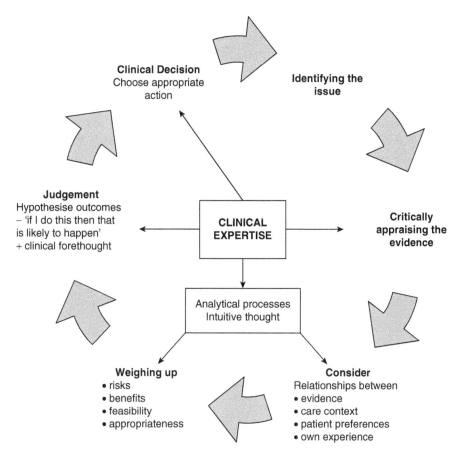

Figure 3.2 Model for clinical decision making

REFLECTIVE PRACTICE

Modern healthcare is often defined in terms of four precepts: that it should be evidence-based; patient-centred and inclusive of carers and the community; continuous and coordinated across settings; and ethically sound and regulated (Petrova et al., 2006). Reflection is a central feature of clinical judgement and decision making as it requires health professionals to consider and make links between the evidence, their own knowledge, skills and experience and that of other team members as well as patient preferences, beliefs and values. However, for this to be effective in aiding clinical judgement it must be undertaken in a clear and structured way rather than simply 'thinking about' the issues. It has been identified that appropriate reflection and particularly reflective writing encourage the transfer of knowledge from one situation to another and help in knowledge transformation – consideration of the relevance current experiences may have for future activities (Nielsen et al., 2007).

Values and personal experience and beliefs influence the way we interpret and apply evidence to support our practice (Fulford et al., 2012). Self-awareness, as reflection and a level of scrutiny and introspection, aligned to the principles of clinical supervision, enables us to examine the motivations and drivers which inform our judgements, bias and attitudes to patients, and care delivery or prioritisation.

The Nursing and Midwifery Council, in the *Future Nurse: Standards of Proficiency for Registered Nurses* document (NMC, 2018a), requires the nurse to: take responsibility for continuous self-reflection, seeking and responding to support and feedback to develop their professional knowledge and skills (p. 9). Furthermore, the NMC (2019) requires five written reflective accounts as part of its revalidation process, encouraging nurses, midwives and nursing associates to reflect on their practice, so they can identify any improvements or changes to their practice as a result of what they have learnt (NMC, 2019). This is based on the assumption that nurses and those that they work with have personal knowledge of what desirable practice means to them individually, and would, if they had the opportunity or the resources, want to work in a particular way. At its simplest, reflection can be described as giving something serious thought or consideration. It involves,

> ... the throwing back of thoughts and memories, in cognitive acts such as thinking, contemplation, meditation and any other form of attentive consideration, in order to make sense of them, and to make contextually appropriate changes if they are required. (Taylor, 2000: 3)

The idea of reflection is centred on the notion that practitioners want to move practice forward and see the benefits in challenging their own practice. Reflective learning is thus a test of their understanding and of the situations in which practice occurs. In this way, reflection is different from simply recalling an event, or even discussing a day at work with a colleague. It is instead an active process requiring the individual to explore things that they may not wholly be comfortable with and to make changes to their practice if need be. It does this by a process of self-exploration, transforming insights and observations gained as part of clinical practice, into knowledge that can be used when making future decisions (Sibson & Riebe, 2016). In this sense, reflection is both a personal and purposeful activity, and refers to the capacity to uncover our assumptions about ourselves, other people, and the workplace.

It is through reflective practice that learning becomes an experimental approach to individualised challenges that in turn form the basis for further exploration and investigation. Reflection helps nurses to understand what they already know (individual); identify what they need to know in order to advance understanding of the subject (contextual); make sense of new information and feedback in the context of their own experience (relational); and guide choices for further learning (developmental). It is not enough just to do, and neither is it enough just to think. Learning from experience must involve links between the doing and the thinking. Reflection has been promoted as a means of accessing this 'theory–practice gap' and provide a foundation on which to develop subsequent knowledge. Learning of this kind is at its best when it emphasises the individual.

The benefits of reflective practice are well recorded and include redefining understanding of professional knowledge; expanding personal knowledge or self-awareness; evaluating appropriateness of actions, and personal and professional growth. Reflection assumes:

- a willingness to learn from what happens in practice;
- being open enough to share elements of practice with other people;
- being motivated enough to 'replay' aspects of clinical practice;
- knowledge for clinical practice can emerge from within, as well outside clinical practice;
- being aware of the conditions necessary for reflection to occur;
- a belief that it is possible to change as a practitioner;
- the ability to describe in detail before analysing practice problems;
- recognising the consequences of reflection;
- the ability to articulate what happens in practice;
- a belief that there is no end point in learning about practice;
- not being defensive about what other people notice about one's practice;
- being courageous enough to act on reflection;
- working out schemes to personally action what has been learned;
- being honest in describing clinical practice to others.

Clinical supervision (Hawkins and Shohet, 2012) also provides a strategy in reducing stress and increasing staff retention, due to the professional and personal demands of a role which is not always about recovery or cure, but about supporting individuals through life-changing experience or towards end of life. Schön's model of reflection, within the context of health and care settings, draws on the knowledge, proficiency and experience of the practitioner and enables them to enhance practice through implicit knowledge (Kinsella, 2010) through two stages: 'reflection in action and reflection on action' (Schön, 1994). These approaches enable the practitioner to reflect on what is occurring now and help facilitate problem solving or recognition of strengths and knowledge in action rather than operating on auto-pilot due to the demands of the role and pressures inherent in practice situations. This helps practitioners and services to identify personal and professional development needs as a team or as individuals to enhance evidence-based practice, impacting on excellence in patient care as well as cost-effectiveness, reputational status and retention of staff. Furthermore, reflection on action following an intervention lends itself to practice development through examination of actions, the impact of these, and other influences at the time of the intervention and how this might be enhanced or delivered differently to increase effectiveness and person-centred care. There are a number of reflective models available to the clinician: see Gibbs' Reflective Cycle (Gibbs, 1988), Kolb's Experiential Learning Cycle (Kolb, 2015) and the Reflect Model (Barksby et al., 2015).

VALUES-BASED DECISION MAKING

Recent scrutiny of the NHS has led to a recognition of the need to reflect on current culture and practice and the revisiting of the values which underpin practice – for example, the Mid Staffordshire NHS Foundation Trust Public Inquiry (Francis, 2013).

Values have a key role in today's health services, in the experiences of people who use services, and in the experiences of their families/carers. Central to this is the understanding that patients are at the core of decision making, not simply passive recipients of care or treatment. A values-based approach to healthcare involves taking into account values as well as the evidence base when making decisions about care. Values-based practice (VBP) has been defined by Fulford (2004: 2) as 'the theory and skills base for effective health care decision making where different (and hence potentially conflicting) values are in play'. This is predicated on the belief that different perspectives need to be respected, especially when dealing with challenging topics.

Values-based practice differs from, while being complementary to, other tools in the toolkit of values-based healthcare, such as ethics and health economic theory, in the emphasis it places on the importance of the diversity of individual values, including the values of clinicians, researchers and managers as well as those of patients and carers, and in relying on a number of elements of good process, in particular specific and learnable clinical skills, to support balanced decision making where values conflict.

Decisions in healthcare are increasingly made against a background of complex and often conflicting values. Conflicting values are values that are in conflict one with another either within a given individual or between different individuals: clinicians, for example, often find there is a conflict between their person-centred values of patient choice and their professional commitment to acting in their patients' best interests. There are many other increasingly 'values complex' areas of healthcare, such as clinical governance, audit, quality assurance, concerns about cost-effectiveness, and the use of quality-of-life and other similar measures in preventive and public health.

Complex values are values that mean different things to different people: 'acting with respect', for example, means different things to people from different cultures, or of different ages, at different historical periods. Balanced decision making means decision making that is based on a balance between the complex and conflicting values of those concerned in a given clinical situation.

The respect for alternative points of view (including the patient's) is seen as an opportunity to open dialogue and positively challenge and reflect on personal, societal and organisational values, attitudes and behaviours, all of which have an impact on the care that we give.

Values-based practice is a partner to evidence-based practice in supporting clinical judgement as we square down in individual cases. Squaring down is the process by which in exercising clinical judgement a skilled clinician focuses progressively on the more relevant information and discards the less relevant information arising from history, examination and investigations (Norcross and Wamplod, 2018). Evidence-based practice is vital to bringing the clinician's focus onto the most likely diagnostic and treatment possibilities; values-based practice is vital to matching those possibilities with the particular circumstances presented by this particular patient in this particular situation.

Activity 3.10

Reflect on how your 'values' impact/might impact on your reading and use of research and evidence as part of your work. Are you values-blind in any way? How do you involve patients in the decision-making process? What governs your clinical practice and decision making? Do you make good decisions? What is the evidence for this?

SHARED DECISION MAKING

Shared decision making (SDM) is the main term used to describe decision making between a professional and a lay person (patient or other service user). Jungermann and Fischer (2005) provide a useful model of understanding the dynamics of this particular joint decision-making situation, focusing particularly on whether or not expert advice is accepted or rejected. They suggest there is an 'informational asymmetry' that characterises expert–non-expert decision-making situations (see Table 3.5).

Table 3.5 Differences in knowledge between advisor and client

Clinician	Patient
1. Generalised knowledge about client's problems.	1. Individual knowledge about personal problem
2. Extensive knowledge about relevant facts	2. Little knowledge about relevant facts
3. Statistical knowledge about goals and values	3. Limited awareness about personal goals and values
4. Professional experience with decision outcomes, coping behaviours, clients' biases	4. Little, if any, experience with problem-related decision consequences, coping possibilities, and judgemental demands
5. Explicit knowledge of decision strategies, implicit decision competence and routines	5. No explicit procedural expertise, implicit (unrelated) competence
6. Professional expertise with client's decision-making behaviour	6. Little, if any, experience with advisor's decision strategies

(Jungermann and Fischer, 2005: 159)

This provides a useful framework of thinking about patient involvement in decision making as it supports the need for good communication with patients and families particularly when making decisions around escalation of treatment and in terms of health education.

The Royal College of Physicians (2019) provides a useful structure to help support both the clinician and patient in decision making:

1. Ensure you have a shared understanding between the clinicians, patient, and those close to the patient of what the problems and issues are.
2. Discuss what the likely outcomes are. Try to help the patient identify which outcomes are most important to them and their family.
3. Be clear about what treatments are being proposed and the evidence for this. If a treatment is not considered sufficiently beneficial to be offered, this will need communicating carefully and compassionately.
4. Agree the proposed treatment plan and care you will be organising, for example treatment on the ward or treatment on intensive care.
5. Include discussion of specific treatments, both that require discussion, e.g. CPR, or are important to the patient.

GROUP DECISION MAKING

Healthcare does not take place in a vacuum but is delivered by a team of professionals and ancillary staff. Many of the decisions made in clinical practice are taken collectively. This brings both advantages and disadvantages. By definition, group decisions are participatory and subject to social influence. Perhaps the greatest advantage is that group members tend to be from different specialties and as such provide more information and knowledge. Implementation of the decision is more effective since the people who are putting the decision into practice have contributed to its formulation and feel an investment in it. The participative nature of group decision making means that it can act as a training ground for junior members of staff to develop the skills of questioning and objective analysis and for senior members of staff to act as role-models. The seven-step model presented below offers a structured approach to group decision making.

1. Identify the decision to be made.
2. Examine the data. Perhaps most importantly, ask what additional information is needed.
3. Establish criteria. Identify the criteria or conditions that would determine whether a chosen solution is successful.
4. Discuss potential solutions based on the available evidence.
5. Evaluate options and select the best one. Remember not everyone will necessarily agree; however, whatever decision is reached should be based on the best evidence at the time.
6. Implement the solution.
7. Monitor and evaluate the outcome.

(Adapted from University of Waterloo, 2015)

Group decisions can also be less efficient that those made by an individual. Group decisions can take longer to reach and there may be conflict between group members as to what to do and what is the best evidence to support a particular approach. One of the biggest disadvantages to such decision making is the phenomenon known as Groupthink. Groupthink was a term first put forward by Irving Jarvis (1972) to describe the situation in which a group makes faulty decisions because group pressures lead to a deterioration of 'mental efficiency, reality testing and moral judgement' (1972: 9). Groupthink occurs when individuals in a group feel under pressure to conform to what seems to be the dominant view of the group, and can lead to the following barriers:

*   incomplete survey of alternatives;
*   incomplete survey of objectives;
*   failure to examine risks of preferred choice;
*   failure to reappraise initially rejected alternatives;
*   poor information search;
*   selective bias in processing information at hand;
*   failure to work out contingency plans;
*   low probability of successful outcome.

COMMUNITIES OF PRACTICE

While the concept of communities of practice has been around for a number of years, the term did not really start to shape until the early 1990s with the work of Lave and Wenger (1991) and is largely based on the idea of learning through apprenticeship and situated learning. Communities of practice can be defined as a

> ... group that coheres through sustained mutual engagement on an indigenous enterprise and creating a common repertoire. (Wenger, 1998: 185–6)

This involves healthcare professionals coming together to discuss their ideas, evidence and decision making as part of clinical practice.

Communities of practice are:

> ... a process of social learning that occurs when people who have a common interest in a subject or area collaborate over an extended period of time, sharing ideas and strategies, determine solutions, and build innovations. (Wenger, 2002: 8)

The latter implies an active process of doing and suggests a willingness on the part of members to share ideas and work together as a team. It is not so much that professionals acquire structures or models to understand the world, but they participate in frameworks that have structure. The idea is centred on the notion that practitioners want to move practice forward and see the benefits of collaboration. Learning is thus a test of commitment and the means by which practitioners determine the adequacy of their understanding and of the situations in which practice occurs. In this way a community of practice is:

> ... an intrinsic condition for the existence of knowledge, not least because it provides the intrinsic support necessary for making sense of its heritage ... the social structure of this practice, its power relations, and its conditions for legitimacy define possibilities for learning. (Lave and Wenger, 1991: 98)

What is often missed is the complexities of such groups in their coming together and the sense in which relationships and understandings are structured by its members, the work itself and the nature of the organisation in which the individual works.

Health professionals inevitably participate in communities of practice by virtue of their day-to-day practice. It is as an active member of the community of practice that nurses learn and build competence (Benner, 1984; Benner et al., 1996). In order to have a community of practice, there needs to exist three core components; these being, domain, community and practice.

- The domain refers to a shared interest between group members, in this case nursing.
- The community is the forum that exists and in which members participate, in this case clinical practice.
- Practice refers to the day-to-day activities that make up the job or role. This is accessed through members sharing stories and experiences, information and knowledge, and challenging the way things are done; this includes problem solving, discussion and a willingness to learn from others and mistakes amongst other things.

When viewed in this way communities of practice are a social instrument to create, share and steward knowledge, including tacit knowledge (knowledge gained from doing the job), for the purpose of moving practice forward. The extent by which a community achieves this depends upon the strength and quality of the relationship between group members; the exchange and use of information and knowledge between its members; the ability of a community to resolve differences and move practice forward; and the ability to care for and look after its members.

Summary

- The complexity of care requires finely honed clinical judgement skills to ensure clinical decision making is of the highest standard.
- Nurses' experiences and perspectives/values have a greater impact on their clinical judgement than scientific evidence.
- Clinical judgement and clinical decision making are closely linked but separate concepts.
- Involvement of service users in the decisions and sound clinical decision making are central to EBP.
- Clinical judgement is seen as the 'art' of nursing and central to clinical expertise and involves the weighing up of options and reaching a decision as to appropriate action.
- Both analytical process and intuitive thinking are central to clinical judgement.

FURTHER READING

Standing, M. (2017) *Clinical Judgement and Decision Making in Nursing* (3rd edn). Transforming Nursing Practice Series. London: Sage.

Woodbridge, K. and Fulford, B. (2004) *Whose Values? A Workbook for Values-based Practice in Mental Health Care*. London: The Sainsbury Centre for Mental Health.

USEFUL WEBLINKS

General Medical Council. 'Working with the Principles and Decision-making Models' explores the complexity of decision making and the need to include the patient and their families to achieve good decisions. www.gmc-uk.org/ethical-guidance/ethical-guidance-for-doctors/treatment-and-care-towards-the-end-of-life/working-with-the-principles-and-decision-making-models

NHS Education for Scotland Effective Practitioner. Clinical Decision Making: a good site in which clinical decision making is explored. www.npc.nhs.uk/evidence/making_decisions_better/making_decisions_better.php

4

Finding the Evidence

Marishona Ortega

Learning Outcomes

By the end of the chapter, you will be able to:

- identify and choose appropriate resources when finding evidence;
- understand the use of keywords, subject headings and other techniques when searching for evidence;
- develop a search strategy to locate relevant literature.

INTRODUCTION

It is important that all nurses and healthcare professionals develop the skills of being able to find, interpret and use up-to-date evidence. Evidence-based practice has been defined as 'the integration of the best research evidence with our clinical expertise and our patient's unique values and circumstances' (Straus et al., 2019: 1).

Searching for the 'best research evidence' is an important skill to develop and, as Greenhalgh (2019) has pointed out, you may be rigorous in critically appraising the evidence but if you are seeking answers from the wrong sources then this is a waste of your time and effort. Most forms of evidence are now available online so an important part of finding evidence is being able to navigate your way through the myriad of resources available. This chapter will introduce you to some of the key aspects related to identifying and choosing appropriate sources of evidence.

WHERE IS THE EVIDENCE?

Evidence can take many forms and this chapter will look at different types of evidence both published and unpublished. The value and **credibility** of each type must be considered when trying to establish if it is going to be useful to you and your professional practice.

Books

Books are often the starting point for many people in their search for evidence and they can offer:

- a general overview on a subject and help you identify key topics that you should be aware of;
- useful background information;
- a comparison of different theories;
- references to other sources of information, which you can follow up.

Books, however, will not be the place to find the latest thinking or research on a topic as the information you find in books can sometimes become dated due to the length of the publishing process. This is when you will need to use journals.

Journals

Journals are published at regular intervals, such as monthly or quarterly, and are a primary means of communicating scholarly activity. They contain a range of articles, from editorials and discussion pieces to case studies and clinical trials, all of which contribute to the evidence base.

Discussion and commentary papers can also be important when considering concepts and theories that are central to a profession's knowledge base or where little is known about a topic. There are many thousands of journals in healthcare, and the information found within them will tend to be more specialised and up-to-date than that found in books.

Many journals provide alerting services, so that you can be informed when new issues arise and thus keep up-to-date with the latest thinking in your field.

Activity 4.1

Find out which journals in your subject area you can access via your health library.
Check whether you can access them in print or online.

Government and policy documents

Government and policy documents can prove a valuable source of information. Most of these can be found via the UK government's website at: www.gov.uk or via individual department sites, e.g. the Department of Health and Social Care at: www.gov.uk/government/organisations/department-of-health-and-social-care.

Repositories

Many universities and research institutes make their research outputs available in an institutional repository, which can hold a wide range of material including preliminary versions of journal articles, data sets, interview records, etc. OpenDOAR (https://v2.sherpa.ac.uk/opendoar) is the quality-assured global directory of academic open access repositories, which allows you to search both for repositories and their contents.

Research in progress

It is also possible to find out about research in progress or the very latest research findings on the following sites:

- National Institute for Health Research's (NIHR) Evidence website provides high-quality summaries of findings from health and care research. It includes short summaries, overviews and themed reviews: https://evidence.nihr.ac.uk
- Be Part of Research – find clinical trials by condition or geographical location: https://bepartofresearch.nihr.ac.uk
- PROSPERO, an international prospective register of systematic reviews in health and social care: www.crd.york.ac.uk/prospero
- EU Clinical Trials Register contains information on clinical trials conducted in the European Union (EU), or the European Economic Area (EEA), which started after May 2004. Please note that the status of studies in Great Britain is no longer updated from January 2021: www.clinicaltrialsregister.eu
- The World Health Organization's International Clinical Trials Registry Platform (ICTRP) is a single point of access to information about ongoing and completed clinical trials from a range of providers from around the world. It also provides links to the full original records: http://trialsearch.who.int
- The US National Library of Medicine maintains clinicaltrials.gov, which includes trials and interventional studies from over 200 countries: https://clinicaltrials.gov

Grey literature

Another important source of evidence is known as **grey literature**. This is literature that has not been formally published, but nevertheless may include useful information. Grey literature can include:

Theses

There are several resources that can be searched for theses and/or dissertations, which are undertaken as part of a course of study for various levels of degree (master's and doctorates):

- EThOS – the UK's national thesis service provided by the British Library holds records of at least 90% of all UK doctoral level theses: https://ethos.bl.uk
- DART-Europe e-theses provides a single European portal for the discovery of electronic theses and dissertations: www.dart-europe.org

- Open Access Dissertation & Theses from over 1,100 colleges, universities and research institutions: https://oatd.org
- Proquest Dissertations & Theses Global is a single repository of graduate dissertations and theses from research institutions in 100 countries (subscription required).

In-house publications

In-house publications might include, for example, leaflets, pamphlets, newsletters and reports. The internet is often a good source for locating these. However, there are some specialist databases that include them:

- HMIC (Health Management and Information Consortium) includes publications from the Department of Health and the King's Fund (subscription required)
- IRIS (Institutional Repository for Information Sharing) is the digital library of World Health Organization publications. Includes technical reports, publications and journal articles: https://apps.who.int/iris
- Open Grey is a multidisciplinary European database, covering science, technology, bio-medical science, economics, social science and humanities: www.opengrey.eu – although please note that this site was archived in 2021 at: https://doi.org/10.17026/dans-xtf-47w5

Conferences

Conference papers and presentations can give you an insight into the cutting edge of research where new theories may be presented before they are published in a journal article; however, they can sometimes be difficult to locate. Some conference papers may be included in subject-specific databases such as MEDLINE or CINAHL, but there are additional resources available:

- Conference Proceedings Citation Index available via Web of Science Core Collection includes global coverage of over 200,000 conferences (subscription required)
- ZeTOC, produced by the British Library, allows you to search for conference papers and set up alerts: https://zetoc.jisc.ac.uk (subscription required)
- Nearly 8 million full text conference papers are indexed on Scopus (subscription required)
- Google Scholar includes conferences from specific publishers: https://scholar.google.co.uk

Pre-prints

Pre-prints are manuscripts that have been made available online before they have been certified by peer review or published in a journal, so should not be relied on to guide clinical practice. There are a number of different sources for finding pre-prints:

- bioRxiv is a free online archive for unpublished pre-prints in the life sciences: www.biorxiv.org
- medRxiv is a free online archive for unpublished pre-prints in the medical, clinical and related health sciences: www.medrxiv.org
- OSF Preprints enables you to search across a range of pre-print servers in a variety of disciplines, including medicine and health sciences: https://osf.io/preprints

Searching the internet

Search engines are designed to find information on the internet, Google being the most popular and well known. Tempting as it may be to search for all your evidence on Google, be aware that not all websites are suitable for finding evidence on which to base your practice. Some information that you find will be well researched and well written, but you may also come across information that is at best misleading, at worst, incorrect. Evidence-based practice is about finding the 'best research evidence' and Google may not help you do this, as there are several potential issues that you need to be aware of:

- It is not sufficiently focused to meet all your needs when looking for evidence. For example, at the time of writing, a search for 'smoking and hypnotherapy' on Google produced 6.5 million results. It would be an immense task to look at every result and would not be a good use of your time as you may find yourself looking at lots of irrelevant and unsuitable information.
- Anyone can publish information on the internet; information you find may be based on insubstantial evidence or may be biased in that it only presents one point of view. You need to have the skills to be able to filter the good sites from the bad.
- Information can be out of date.
- You may miss out on finding the latest research as this information may only be available from specialist websites or databases that require a subscription.

It is essential that you do not rely solely on general search engines such as Google and that you instead familiarise yourself with, and use, those that are specifically aimed at nurses and other healthcare professions. See Box 4.1 for examples of suggested search engines.

Box 4.1   Suggested search engines

1. NICE Evidence: a unique source of authoritative, evidence-based information from hundreds of trustworthy and accredited sources. Brings together evidence on health, drugs and technologies, public health, social care, and healthcare management and commissioning in one place. Health and social care staff in England can also access a range of journals and databases (requires an NHS OpenAthens account): www.evidence.nhs.uk
2. SUMSearch 2: simultaneously searches for original studies, systematic reviews, and practice guidelines from PubMed: http://sumsearch.org
3. TRIP: a clinical search engine containing high-quality evidence-based health information to support practice and/or care: www.tripdatabase.com

---

Activity 4.2

Choose and locate one of the search engines identified in Box 4.1. Search for an area of practice that you would like to know more about. How many 'hits' are identified? Consider whether the results are sufficiently focused to meet your needs in searching for evidence.

WHAT RESOURCES ARE AVAILABLE TO HELP WITH EBP?

With the explosion of information and knowledge available on which to base practice, busy practitioners can find themselves overwhelmed. For example, the database MEDLINE contains over 28 million citations with nearly 1 million records added in 2020 alone (US National Library of Medicine, 2020, 2021). There is also a need to ensure that you find the best evidence in relation to your area of interest – not all literature is good evidence and you need to learn to identify the strengths, limitations and applicability to your question of any evidence you find, which is where the skills of **critical appraisal** are required (see Part II of this book). Over the last two decades, various hierarchies of pre-appraised evidence have been developed and have evolved as new resources and services become available. The most recent iteration is Alper and Haynes's (2016) Evidence-Based Health Care (EBHC) Pyramid 5.0, where five categories of resources have been identified and prioritised to help practitioners find appropriate evidence to use when making decisions about care delivery. Starting at the top of the hierarchy, the five levels are:

1. Systems.
2. Synthesised summaries for clinical reference.
3. Systematically derived recommendations (guidelines).
4. Systematic reviews.
5. Studies.

Each level builds systematically on information from the lower levels to 'provide substantially more useful information for guiding clinical decision-making' (Alper and Haynes, 2016: 124).

Systems are computerised or clinical decision support systems (CDSS) which can aid clinical decision-making at the point of care by integrating and summarising all available and appropriate evidence related to a particular clinical issue. An example of a CDSS is the NHS Pathways telephone triage system, which supports the remote assessment of callers to urgent and emergency services (NHS Digital, 2021). According to Sutton et al. (2020), CDSS have evolved since their first use in the 1980s but they are not without their drawbacks.

If a system is not available, the next level down the hierarchy is to look for *synthesised summaries for clinical reference*, which integrate the three lower layers of the hierarchy and include online clinical textbooks. These texts provide an evidence-based summary of best practice at the point of care, which are regularly updated.

Examples include:

- BMJ Best Practice: https://bestpractice.bmj.com/info (available to all the NHS workforce in England)
- Dynamed: www.dynamed.com
- Essential Evidence Plus: www.essentialevidenceplus.com
- UptoDate: www.uptodate.com

Systematically derived recommendations (guidelines) are similar to synthesised summaries but will generally focus on a single condition or disease such as the assessment and management of bipolar disorder.

Providers include:

- National Institute for Health & Care Excellence (NICE) guidelines: www.nice.org.uk/guidance
- Scottish Intercollegiate Guidelines Network (SIGN) guidelines: www.sign.ac.uk
- Profession-specific guidance produced by organisations or charities

Systematic reviews provide rigorous reviews of evidence relating to specific areas of interest and are also advocated as high-quality sources of information. Individual reviews can be found in several resources including:

- Cochrane Database of Systematic Reviews, which focuses on the effectiveness of healthcare interventions: www.cochranelibrary.com
- *Campbell Systematic Reviews*: open access journal, produced by the Campbell Collaboration, which focuses on ageing, crime and justice, disability, education, nutrition and social welfare: https://onlinelibrary.wiley.com/journal/18911803
- *JBI Evidence Synthesis*, an international, peer-reviewed online journal produced by JBI (formerly Joanna Briggs Institute) which publishes systematic and scoping reviews (and protocols): https://journals.lww.com/jbisrir

Alper and Haynes also suggest that guidelines, systematic reviews and studies should be subdivided into filtered (pre-appraised) and synopses (appraised and extracted) which means that you don't need to assess the quality yourself. The following resources may also prove useful:

- EvidenceAlerts is a continuously updated repository of current best evidence from research to support evidence-based clinical decisions. www.evidencealerts.com
- Evidence-based abstraction journals such as:
  - *Evidence-Based Nursing*: http://ebn.bmj.com
  - *Evidence-Based Mental Health*: http://ebmh.bmj.com
  - *Evidence-Based Medicine*: https://ebm.bmj.com
  - *ACP Journal Club*: http://annals.org/aim/journal-club

However, if your area of interest is not covered by any of the resources listed above, then your ultimate source will be original *studies*, which you will need to appraise to identify their strengths, limitations and applicability to your question. This is where you will need to develop your skills in searching for evidence.

SEARCHING FOR EVIDENCE

Searching for evidence or literature searching is a skill that takes time and practice to develop. Many of the resources discussed below will have online tutorials that guide you through the steps you need to take to make best use of them and it is well worth spending some time working through these. Your health librarian will also be able to help you develop the skills that you need, so it is advisable to book an appointment to see them individually or attend a training session. It will be time well spent and save you a great deal of effort and frustration later when you are searching for evidence to support your practice.

There are a number of steps to follow when searching for evidence (overviewed in Figure 4.1).

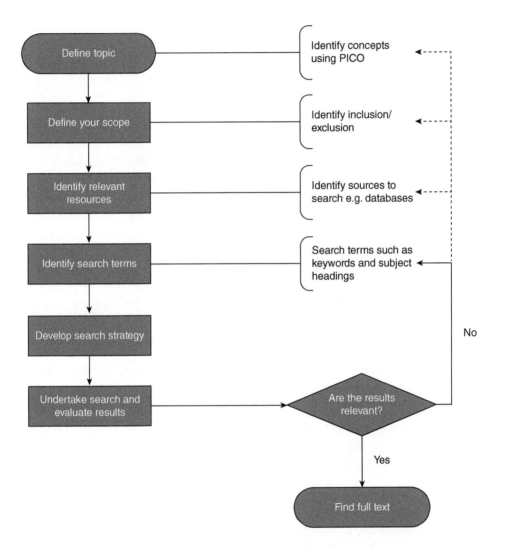

Figure 4.1   Flowchart showing the steps of searching for evidence

Define your topic

Although it is tempting to start searching straightaway, it is a good idea to plan your search by defining your topic, which starts with a focused research question. Without this, it can be very difficult and time consuming to identify appropriate resources and search for relevant evidence. A focused research question will ensure that your search is also focused, which will hopefully mean that you do not retrieve lots of irrelevant results.

A good way to create a focused question and to structure your search is to use the **PICO** model, which is ideal for clinical questions where a healthcare intervention is involved (Richardson et al., 1995). The terms you identify using PICO will form the main concepts of your **search strategy** and will help ensure that your search is focused.

P = Patient, problem or population – who are the people that you are interested in? Do they have similar characteristics, i.e. age, ethnicity or disease/condition?

I = Intervention – how are you considering intervening – drugs, surgery, etc.?

C = Comparison – is there an alternative that you wish to compare? This could be comparing two different types of interventions or comparing an intervention against no intervention.

O = Outcome – what is the effect of the intervention? This could be a reduction in symptoms, benefits or improved prognosis, e.g. smoking cessation.

For example, if PICO was applied to the question 'What is the effectiveness of hypno-therapy compared to nicotine replacement therapy for helping people to quit smoking?' it would look like Table 4.1.

Table 4.1   Main concepts of a search strategy using PICO

Patient/problem	Intervention	Comparison	Outcome
Smokers	Hypnotherapy	Nicotine replacement therapy	Smoking cessation

There are many other frameworks that can help you create a focused literature search. These are just a few:

- PICOC – **P**opulation, **I**ntervention, **C**omparison, **O**utcome, **C**ontext (Petticrew and Roberts, 2006);
- PEO – **P**opulation, **E**xposure, **O**utcome – useful for qualitative research (Moola et al., 2015);
- ECLIPSE – **E**xpectation, **C**lient group, **L**ocation, **I**mpact, **P**rofessionals, **S**ervice – useful for health policy/management topics (Wildridge and Bell, 2002);
- SPICE – **S**etting, **P**erspective, **I**ntervention, **C**omparison, **E**valuation – useful for qualitative research topics or the social sciences (Booth, 2004);
- SPIDER – **S**ample, **P**henomenon of **I**nterest, **D**esign, **E**valuation, **R**esearch type – useful for qualitative and **mixed methods** studies (Cooke et al., 2012).

Select an area that you would like to know more about and identify the Patient/problem, Intervention, Comparison and Outcome (PICO) using the form in Appendix 2.

Activity 4.3

Define your scope

It is also a good idea to define the scope of your search. This is where you can consider any *inclusion* or *exclusion criteria*, which will help focus your search by increasing the likelihood of retrieving literature relevant to your topic or question. Inclusion and exclusion criteria are the factors that you can use to limit the results of your search by deciding which articles should be included or excluded. These factors can include publication date, language, study design and geographic location to name but a few.

Examples of inclusion criteria:

- published in the English language;
- published in the last five years;
- published in a peer-reviewed journal

Examples of exclusion criteria:

- published in a non-English language;
- published over five years ago;
- published in a non-peer-reviewed journal.

Activity 4.4

Define the scope of your PICO question in Appendix 2 – do you want to limit your search in any way?

Identify relevant resources to search

To ensure that you are aware of what is available on a given topic and access the most up-to-date information, you will need to search databases. Databases contain records of journal articles, dissertations, book chapters, reviews, etc. often in a specific subject area. They enable users to search for information by keywords, subject headings and descriptors, and will sometimes provide full text access to the journal articles in question.

The databases that are of interest here are those related to the healthcare professions, and some suggested databases are listed in Box 4.2. The ones most commonly used by nurses and healthcare professionals are CINAHL (Cumulative Index to Nursing and Allied Health Literature) and MEDLINE. CINAHL is one of the most comprehensive databases for nurses and allied health professions. It indexes over 3,000 peer-reviewed journals (EBSCO, 2021). There are five different versions of CINAHL, including CINAHL Plus, CINAHL with Full Text and CINAHL Complete, which offers maximum journal and full text coverage. Access is via subscription only and therefore it will depend upon what your library subscribes to as to what will be available to you.

MEDLINE is produced by the United States National Library of Medicine and contains more than 28 million citations from over 5,200 journals in 40 languages (US National Library of Medicine, 2021). Although the majority of journals indexed are medical, it also indexes a number of nursing journals. There are various online versions of MEDLINE and it can be freely accessed using PubMed.

There are a number of information service providers, through which education and health communities can access a range of databases and support services from one platform. Examples include Ovid and EBSCOhost. Many service providers allow you to search across multiple databases, which will help save you time and effort.

Although the search interfaces from different providers may differ slightly, the principles of searching will be the same. Most will offer both basic and advanced searching as well as allowing you to combine and save searches. However, the easiest way to learn how to get the most out of searching the databases available to you is by booking a training session with your health librarian or by working through the online tutorials for each database.

Box 4.2   Suggested databases

AMED: allied and complementary medicine database. Includes citations from over 500 journals related to allied health professions, complementary medicine and palliative care (subscription required).

APA PsycINFO: is the largest resource devoted to peer-reviewed literature in mental health and behavioural sciences. Compiled by the American Psychological Association it includes journal articles, books, book chapters and dissertations (subscription required).

BNI (British Nursing Index): UK nursing and midwifery database indexes the most popular English language nursing journals published primarily in the UK, with a small selection of titles from the US and Australia (subscription required).

CINAHL (Cumulative Index to Nursing and Allied Health Literature): literature relating to nursing and allied health professions from over 3,000 peer-reviewed journals (subscription required).

Cochrane Library: is a collection of databases that contain different types of high-quality, independent evidence to inform healthcare decision making. This includes the Cochrane Database of Systematic Reviews, which contains full text systematic reviews, Cochrane Central Register of Controlled Trials (CENTRAL), which provides reports of randomised and quasi-randomised controlled trials, and Cochrane Clinical Answers: www.cochranelibrary.com

EMBASE (Excerpta Medica): an international biomedical database, similar to MEDLINE but having a greater focus on drugs and pharmacology (subscription required).

Global Index Medicus: maintained by the World Health Organization and brings together WHO's regional databases that cover biomedical and public health issues, including the African Index Medicus (AIM), the Scientific and Technical

(Continued)

Literature of Latin America and the Caribbean (LILACS), the Index Medicus for the Eastern Mediterranean Region (IMEMR) and the Index Medicus for South-East Asia Region (IMSEAR) and the Western Pacific Region Index Medicus (WPRIM): www.globalindexmedicus.net

MEDLINE: the primary source for biomedical data from 1966 to the present. Compiled by the US National Library of Medicine (subscription required).

MIDIRS Reference Database: over 400 journals and other resources related to midwifery (subscription required).

PEDro (Physiotherapy Evidence Database): a free database of over 50,000 trials, reviews and guidelines in physiotherapy: https://pedro.org.au

OTSeeker: a database that contains abstracts of systematic reviews, randomised controlled trials and other resources relevant to occupational therapy interventions. Please note that due to a lack of funding, content from 2016 onwards is not comprehensive: www.otseeker.com

PubMed: provides free web access to MEDLINE and contains more than 30 million records for biomedical literature, life science journals and online books. Records may include links to full text content from PubMed Central or publisher websites: https://pubmed.ncbi.nlm.nih.gov

ScienceDirect: full text access to 4,000 journals and over 30,000 books from the scientific, technical and health disciplines published by Elsevier (subscription required).

Social Care Online: a free database provided by the Social Care Institute for Excellence (SCIE). Includes legislation, government documents, practice and guidance, systematic reviews, research briefings, reports, journal articles and websites: www.scie-socialcareonline.org.uk

SCOPUS: the largest abstract and citation database of peer-reviewed literature: scientific journals, books and conference proceedings. Contains nearly 80 million records from over 24,000 journals (subscription required).

Web of Science: a collection of databases in the fields of science, social sciences, arts and humanities. Includes conference proceedings (subscription required).

Activity 4.5

Find out which databases you can access via your library.

Look at your completed PICO question in Appendix 2 and list which databases are relevant to your search.

Databases generally store publication information in the form of article title, author(s), journal title, year, volume, issue and page numbers. Many will include an abstract, which is a short summary of the content of the article. Reading the abstract as well as the title will help you determine whether the article will be relevant to you. Figure 4.2 is an example of a record from PubMed.

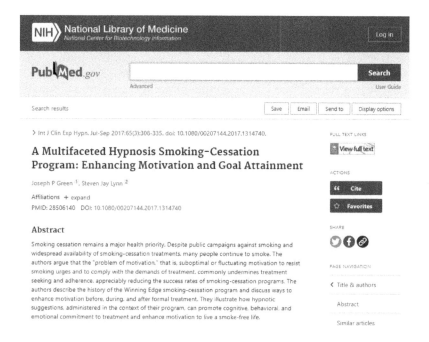

Figure 4.2 Example of a PubMed record

Available at: https://pubmed.ncbi.nlm.nih.gov/28506140/ (accessed 4 August 2021).

Identify search terms

Having used PICO to identify the main concepts of your search, you should also consider and note:

- synonyms – words or phrases that share the same meaning, e.g. heart attack and myocardial infarction;
- acronyms/abbreviations – where phrases have been shortened to a set of letters, e.g. CBT and cognitive behavioural therapy;
- alternative spellings, e.g. paediatrics and pediatrics;
- alternative terms, e.g. learning disabilities and learning disorders.

These will form the keywords that you will use in your search strategy.

Table 4.2 shows some possible alternative terms for our question: 'What is the effectiveness of hypnotherapy compared to nicotine replacement therapy for helping people to quit smoking?'

Look at the concepts you have identified in your PICO question in Appendix 2 and consider what other terms may be associated with them. You may have come up with a long list or just a few phrases. Whichever is the case, these are your keywords and will form part of your search strategy.

Develop a search strategy

A search strategy is the information (keywords, etc.) that you enter into the database to find the evidence that you want. These can be simple or complex – you will see in Chapter 8 that extensive searches are used in systematic reviews.

Table 4.2 Main concepts of a search strategy including a selection of alternative terms

Patient/problem	Intervention	Comparison	Outcome
Smoker	Hypnotherapy	Nicotine replacement	Smoking cessation
Smokers	Hypnosis	therapy	Tobacco use cessation
Smoking		NRT	Quit smoking
Tobacco use			
Cigarettes			
Cigars			

Boolean operators

These are the words 'AND', 'OR' and 'NOT' which are used to combine search terms. For example, if you are interested in the effect hypnotherapy has on smoking, you may consider using the keywords smoking AND hypnotherapy. A search of PubMed using Boolean operators generated the following results:

Smoking **AND** Hypnotherapy – 292 articles containing both words.

'AND' narrows your search by only retrieving articles where both terms are present.

Smoking **OR** Hypnotherapy – 344,339 articles containing either of the terms.

'OR' broadens your search by retrieving either term; this is useful where there are alternative terms for a concept that you wish to include in your strategy.

Smoking **NOT** Hypnotherapy – 328,764 articles containing Smoking but not Hypnotherapy.

'NOT' should be used with caution in that you may exclude relevant articles that happen to mention the excluded term.

Table 4.3 Example of combining search terms using Boolean operators

Patient/problem		Intervention		Comparison		Outcome
Smoker	**AND**	Hypnotherapy	**AND**	Nicotine	**AND**	Smoking cessation
OR		**OR**		replacement		**OR**
Smokers		Hypnosis		therapy		Tobacco use cessation
OR				**OR**		**OR**
Smoking				NRT		Quit smoking
OR						
Tobacco use						
OR						
Cigarettes						
OR						
Cigars						

Table 4.3 includes Boolean operators to combine your search terms. This information can then be converted into your search strategy:

1. Smoker
2. Smokers
3. Smoking
4. Tobacco use
5. Cigarettes
6. Cigars
7. 1 OR 2 OR 3 OR 4 OR 5 OR 6
8. Hypnotherapy
9. Hypnosis
10. 8 OR 9
11. Nicotine replacement therapy
12. NRT
13. 11 OR 12
14. Smoking cessation
15. Tobacco use cessation
16. Quit smoking
17. 14 OR 15 OR 16
18. 7 AND 10 AND 13 AND 17

Figure 4.3 shows what the strategy looks like in PubMed.

Type the keywords you identified earlier into a database of your choice and combine using Boolean operators. Note how many articles are retrieved.

Activity 4.7

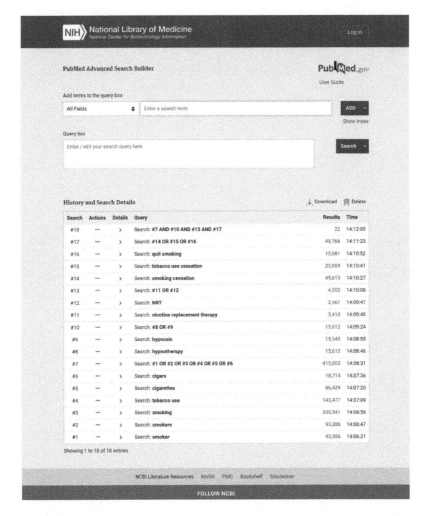

Figure 4.3   Example of a search using PubMed Advanced Search Builder using Boolean operators

Available at: https://pubmed.ncbi.nlm.nih.gov/advanced/ (accessed 1 September 2021).

Truncation

Truncation allows you to search for variations of words without having to include them all in your search strategy. A truncation mark (usually an asterisk * or dollar sign $ – check the database help guide as to which symbol should be used) put after a word-stem allows you to search for all the variations.

For example, PubMed uses an asterisk * as truncation, so rather than searching for:

- Smoker
- Smokers
- Smoking

you could simply put smok* and this will retrieve all the variations. This method can save you time when searching but it is important to be aware that this type of searching can generate lots of results as any passing reference to the word is retrieved. Consideration also needs to be given as to where to truncate words; for example, when searching PubMed for hypno* nearly 145,000 records were retrieved, but in addition to articles about hypnotherapy or hypnosis, it also included articles about hypnotic drugs and hypnosedatives, which would not be relevant to the search.

Phrase searching

In addition to searching for individual keywords, it is also possible to search for phrases by putting quotation marks (" ") around the terms, e.g. "nicotine replacement therapy", which means only records containing that exact phrase will be retrieved.

Wildcards

Where words may have alternative spellings – such as paediatrics and pediatrics – a symbol (often a question mark ? or hash symbol # – check the database help guide as to which symbol should be used) can be placed within the word at the point where the variation may occur. In this example you would use 'p?ediatrics' to ensure words with either the UK or American spelling will be then searched for and retrieved.

Adjacency operators

Many databases will allow you to search for a word within a specified number of another word of your choice, which can be helpful if there isn't a phrase search is not appropriate. For example, in the EBSCOhost interface, 'nicotine N2 replacement' will find the word nicotine within two words of replacement (regardless of the order in which they appear). These are called adjacency or proximity operators and they will generally differ between databases so it is advisable to check the online help.

Field searching

One technique to increase the precision of your search is to restrict your search for keywords to specific fields of an article record, e.g. title or abstract. This means that results will only be retrieved where your specific keyword is in a specific field.

Subject headings

Many databases use a controlled vocabulary to describe and index the content of articles, with the most well known being Medical Subject Headings commonly known as **MeSH**, which is used in both MEDLINE and the Cochrane Library. CINAHL currently has over 16,000 subject headings (EBSCO Connect, 2021), which are based on MeSH but with additional specific nursing and allied health headings added as appropriate. Subject headings are usually updated annually to reflect new developments; for example, new subject headings for COVID-19 were created in both MEDLINE and CINAHL in 2020. The subject headings in these databases are hierarchical and it is possible to 'explode' a heading to retrieve all references indexed with that heading as well as all references indexed with any narrower subject heading.

Using subject headings combined with your keywords (using the Boolean OR operator) is a good way to ensure you are retrieving all relevant articles. Look for a link within the database that will take you to their subject headings, so that you can either browse or search them. MeSH is freely available to browse at: www.nlm.nih.gov/mesh

As can be seen in Figure 4.4, the recommended MeSH term for nicotine replacement products is 'Tobacco Use Cessation Devices'. Subject headings can be included alongside your keywords in your search strategy.

An example of a search strategy using truncation, phrase searching and MeSH headings:

1. Smok*
2. Tobacco use
3. Cigar*
4. Smoking [MeSH Terms]
5. Tobacco smoking [MeSH Terms]
6. Cigarette smoking [MeSH Terms]
7. Cigar smoking [MeSH Terms]
8. 1 OR 2 OR 3 OR 4 OR 5 OR 6 OR 7
9. Hypnotherapy
10. Hypnosis
11. Hypnosis [MeSH Terms]
12. 9 OR 10 OR 11
13. "Nicotine replacement therapy"

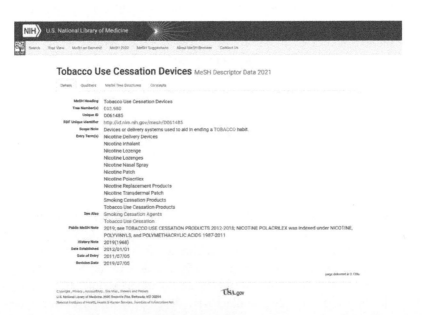

Figure 4.4   An extract for the entry in MeSH for tobacco use cessation devices

Available at: meshb.nlm.nih.gov/record/ui?ui=D061485 (accessed 4 August 2021).

14. NRT
15. Tobacco Use Cessation Devices [MeSH Terms]
16. 13 OR 14 OR 15
17. "Smoking cessation"
18. "Tobacco use cessation"
19. "Quit smoking"
20. Smoking Cessation [MeSH Terms]
21. Tobacco Use Cessation [MeSH Terms]
22. 17 OR 18 OR 19 OR 20 OR 21
23. 8 AND 12 AND 16 AND 22

This strategy would retrieve articles potentially relevant to the original question: 'What is the effectiveness of hypnotherapy compared to nicotine replacement therapy for helping people to quit smoking?'

Figure 4.5 shows how the search strategy would look in PubMed.

> Search the subject headings of your chosen database and check whether there are any associated with your keywords. Include these in your search strategy. Note how many articles are retrieved and compare this to your earlier search.
>
> **Activity 4.8**

Limiting

Most databases allow you to limit your search in certain ways once your keywords and/or subject headings have been entered. This is where it is possible to limit your search according to your inclusion/exclusion criteria, which were identified as part of the planning process. For example, you may choose to limit by publication date – choosing a particular year or span of years. This can be useful if you are interested in the most recent information about a topic. Other limits include language – you may choose to retrieve only English language articles; or patient group, which would include child, adult, etc. Some databases may allow you to limit your search to particular types of evidence – research papers, reviews, meta-analyses, etc.

Undertake search and evaluate results

It is important that when undertaking a search for evidence that you evaluate the results that are retrieved. You may not always be able to tell from an article title as to whether it is relevant to your question. Therefore, it is a good idea to also look at the abstract of the article, which will provide a short summary of the content. If you find that you have too many results, even after limiting your search by your inclusion criteria, then you may need to re-assess either your search strategy, the question that you are answering or both. Consider whether your search terms are too broad or whether the question is not focused enough.

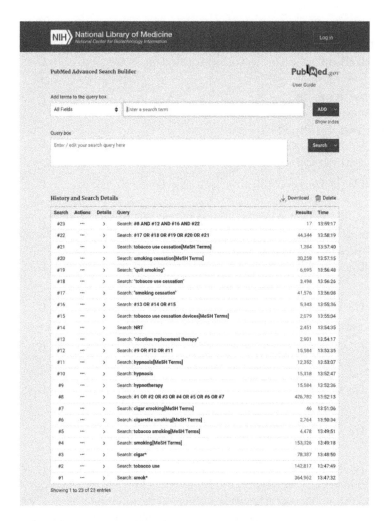

Figure 4.5   Example of a search using PubMed Advanced Search Builder using truncation, phrase searching and MeSH headings

Available at: www.ncbi.nlm.nih.gov/pubmed (accessed 1 September 2021).

Searching for evidence is an iterative process requiring continual review and refinement in order to develop an optimal search, which locates all relevant literature but ensures that you are not overwhelmed with irrelevant results. Remember that your health librarian can help you if you need further assistance.

Find full text

Once you have a list of results that are relevant to your question, the next step is to find the full text of the articles. Many databases will include links to the full text where it is available to you. If the full text is not available, remember that most libraries will offer an

Inter-Library Loan or Document Supply service, whereby they are able to obtain journal articles (as well as books and other material) for you from other libraries, including the British Library. Contact your library for more details, including charges.

In recent years there has been a growth in 'open access' publishing, where research findings are made freely available. Databases such as the Directory of Open Access Journals provide information from nearly 17,000 open access journals (available at: https://doaj.org).

ADDITIONAL SEARCHING TECHNIQUES

Citation pearl growing

Beyond browsing MeSH, there is an additional method of identifying search terms, known as **citation pearl growing**. This is where an article that exactly matches your criteria is located (the pearl) and it is then scanned to locate subject headings or other relevant keywords. These new terms can then be included in your search strategy.

Related articles

Many databases, including PubMed, provide links to 'related articles', which will allow you to access articles on a similar subject. This can be useful in tracking down further relevant articles; however, it must be used with care as it is very easy to get side-tracked into areas that are related to, but not specifically about your chosen topic.

Author searching

In addition to searching by keyword or subject heading, most databases also give you the option of searching by authors' names. You may be aware that a particular author has written extensively on a topic. If so, you may want to search for literature written by that individual as this may lead you to other relevant articles.

Hand searching

You may find when looking through the results of your search that many relevant articles are published in one or two journals. Therefore, it may be useful to undertake a hand search of these journals, that is systematically (i.e. by hand) searching through each issue of the journal within your selected date range, to identify relevant literature. Although time-intensive, hand searching can be a useful technique to identify articles that may not have been indexed correctly by a database.

Reference list searching

The reference lists of relevant articles can also be scanned to identify other further articles of interest.

MANAGING YOUR REFERENCES

Most databases include the facility to save searches, save, print or email links to articles as well as export results to reference management software such as EndNote or RefWorks. This software can help you keep track of useful references as well as create reference lists or bibliographies in different referencing styles such as Harvard or Vancouver. If your library doesn't subscribe to this software, there are freely available tools such as Zotero (www. zotero.org) and Mendeley (www.mendeley.com) that you can use to manage and store your references.

STEPS TO SUCCESS

When searching for literature there are a few simple steps that will help you with the process:

- Find out which databases are provided by your library.
- Familiarise yourself with the databases and how they work – what subject headings, truncation and wildcard symbols, etc. are used in each.
- When identifying your search terms be precise about what it is you want to find.
- Remember that your search terms can be combined using Boolean operators to build a search strategy.
- Limit your search as appropriate, e.g. by date, language or study type.
- Evaluate the results and refine your search as necessary.
- If you need help, remember that your health librarian can assist you with finding the best available evidence.

Activity 4.9

Having completed the 'Formulating a Question and Searching for Evidence' template in Appendix 2, try out your search on one of the databases and evaluate the results. Reflect on your learning and identify areas where your searching skills need to improve.

Summary

- There are resources available to help you integrate evidence into practice - systems, synthesised summaries for clinical reference, systematically derived recommendations (guidelines) and systematic reviews.
- The key to finding evidence is having a clear and focused question. The PICO model or, depending on your topic, one of the other models can be used in this process.

- It is important to be aware of what resources are relevant on your subject and available to you when searching for evidence.
- Many databases use a controlled vocabulary (subject headings) to describe and index the content of articles, e.g. MeSH. Combining keywords with subject headings using Boolean operators can provide the means to locating relevant literature.
- Techniques such as using truncation or wildcards can help streamline your search.
- Searching for evidence is a skill that takes time and practice to develop and librarians are a key resource in helping you find the information that you need.

FURTHER READING

Aveyard, H. and Sharp, P. (2017) *A Beginner's Guide to Evidence Based Practice in Health and Social Care* (3rd edn). London: Open University Press/McGraw Hill Education.

Bettany-Saltikov, J. and McSherry, R. (2016) *How to do a Systematic Literature Review in Nursing: A Step-by-Step Guide* (2nd edn). London: Open University Press/McGraw Hill Education.

Booth, A., Sutton, A. and Papaioannou, D. (2016) *Systematic Approaches to a Successful Literature Review* (2nd edn). London: Sage.

Czaplewski, L.M. (2012) 'Searching the literature: a researcher's perspective', *Journal of Infusion Nursing*, 35(1): 20–6.

Fowler, J. (2020) 'From staff nurse to nurse consultant: Academic essays part 5: literature searching', *British Journal of Nursing*, 29(20): 1215.

Gerrish, K. and Lathlean, J. (eds) (2015) *The Research Process in Nursing* (7th edn). Oxford: Wiley Blackwell.

Greenhalgh, T. (2019) *How to Read a Paper: The Basics of Evidence-Based Medicine and Healthcare* (6th edn). Oxford: John Wiley & Sons.

Jameson, J. and Walsh, M.E. (2017) 'Tools for evidence-based vascular nursing practice: achieving information literacy for lifelong learning', *Journal of Vascular Nursing*, 35(4): 201–10.

Moule, P. (2021) *Making Sense of Research in Nursing, Health and Social Care* (7th edn). London: Sage.

Moule, P., Aveyard, H. and Goodman, M. (2017) *Nursing Research: An Introduction* (3rd edn). London: Sage.

Stillwell, S.B., Fineout-Overholt, E., Melnyk, B.M. and Williamson, K.M. (2010) 'Evidence-based practice, step by step: searching for the evidence', *American Journal of Nursing*, 110(5): 41–7.

Conclusion to Part I

The aim of this section was to provide you with an underpinning knowledge of the various aspects of evidence-based practice and the skills associated with the first four aspects of the process as identified in Chapter 1. That is:

- the ability to identify what counts as appropriate evidence;
- forming a question to enable you to find evidence for consideration;
- developing a search strategy;
- finding the evidence.

This section ends with a crossword puzzle, with clues to answers relevant to Chapters 1 to 4. The answers can be found on p. **218**.

CROSSWORD PUZZLE

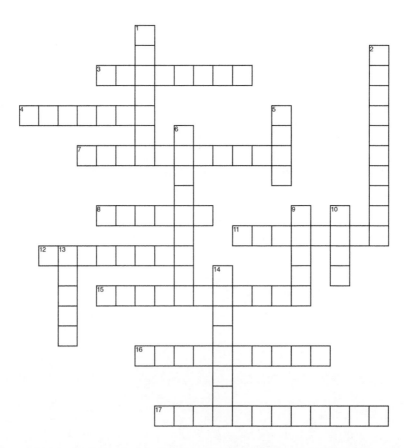

Across

3. Information on which to base best practice (8)

4. Words used to combine search terms (7)

7. Items of evidence grouped together to provide a greater effect (11)

8. Theorist's surname – proposed a framework of nursing knowledge (6)

11. Set of logically connected ideas (8)

12. Central point for storing information in relation to specific topics (8)

15. Considering implications of decisions over time (11)

16. Belief that only what can be observed can be called fact (10)

17. Belief that humans actively construct their reality (12)

Down

1. A body of knowledge organised in a systematic way (7)

2. The belief that reality is ordered and can be studied objectively (10)

5. Terms used to describe medical subject headings (4)

6. Essential aspect of clinical decision making (9)

9. Knowledge used by practitioners drawn from experience (5)

10. Format for creating search questions (4)

13. Process for gathering information to promote effective care (5)

14. Last name of the 'father' of EBM (8)

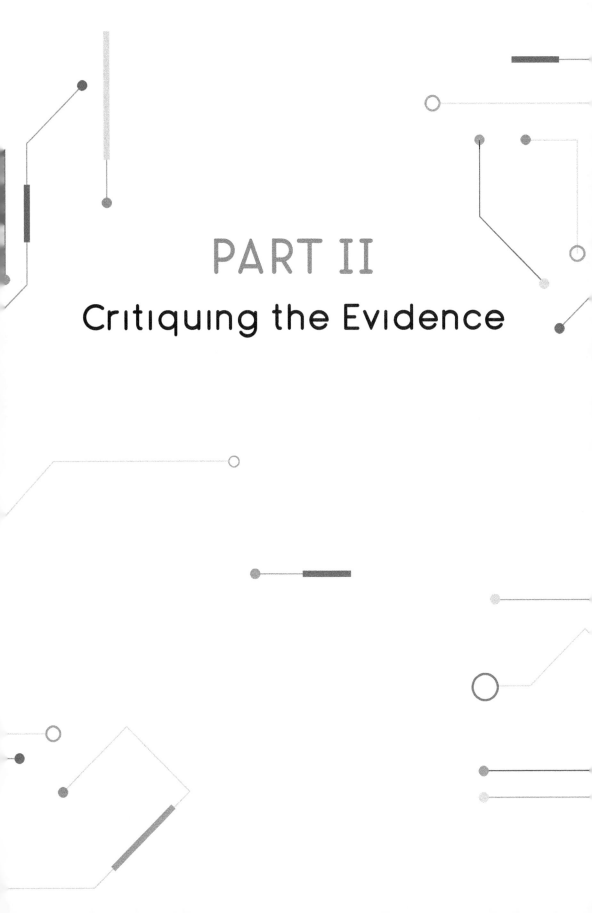

PART II
Critiquing the Evidence

5

What is Critical Appraisal?

Paul Linsley and Ros Kane

Learning Outcomes

By the end of the chapter, you will be able to:

- define critical appraisal and its role in evidence-based practice (EBP);
- discuss the steps required for critical appraisal in relation to different forms of evidence;
- understand the skills of critical appraisal;
- locate appropriate critical appraisal tools.

INTRODUCTION

Critical appraisal essentially means the assessment of the quality of a piece of research. Furthermore, it is the 'process of systematically examining research evidence to assess its validity, results and relevance before using it to inform a decision' and is 'an essential part of evidence-based clinical practice that includes the process of systematically finding, appraising and acting on evidence of effectiveness' (Hill and Spittlehouse, 2001: 1). It is important that nurses and other healthcare professionals critically appraise all evidence before integrating it into practice, to ensure its worth and value to their patients.

In order to determine what is the 'best' evidence, we need a means by which to critically appraise research so that we can make use of it as part of our clinical practice. The aim of this chapter is to provide a robust and simple approach for assessing the value and credibility of research and its usefulness to clinical practice. Examples of critical appraisal tools are included in order to help you structure your approach to reading and critiquing a research paper. The skills needed to undertake a critical appraisal are outlined and explored.

WHAT IS CRITICAL APPRAISAL?

The critical in critical appraisal 'means the objective analysis and evaluation of an issue in order to form a judgement' and appraisal 'is the act of assessing the worth value or quality of the thing' (*Oxford English Dictionary*, 2021). Critical appraisal is essentially the assessment of the usefulness of evidence, meaning its quality and its applicability to context.

When we first think about critical appraisal there is a tendency to think that it is all about looking for problems in a research paper – the things that might make us question the study's conclusions, or to lack confidence in them. It is not only about identifying weaknesses in a piece of evidence but also about noting the strengths – critical appraisal should be an objective consideration of the merits and limitations of the evidence. It's about looking for the positives – those things that give us confidence that a study has been well-designed and executed and consider its relevance to our clinical practice.

One of the problems with published work is people assume that because something is in print it must be high-quality evidence, but this may not always be the case. Although most research papers are subject to a rigorous peer review process – where experts have scrutinised the work and commented on its appropriateness for publication – not all published work is necessarily always of a high standard. Even when research is of high quality, most studies will still have some methodological weaknesses, as Nieswiadomy and Bailey (2017) identified; there is no such thing as a perfect research study, all have flaws or limitations of some sort. If research findings are to be used in practice it is vital those implementing them are aware of these limitations and consider their implications.

Issues related to the **validity**, **reliability**, **trustworthiness** and **relevance** of research studies are of prime importance to critical appraisal (Polit and Beck, 2018) and all these concepts will be considered in more depth in later chapters. Briefly, however, validity relates to whether or not the claims made in a study are accurate; so, for instance, if the paper suggests its findings are generalisable, there is a need to consider if the methodology used supports such a claim. Reliability is concerned with identifying if the results are dependable and replicable and involves asking the question, 'If the research was repeated would the same results be found?' The concept of trustworthiness relates to whether data can be considered objective and credible. Finally, relevance is seen as a consideration as to whether the findings can be applied to the practice setting.

Although these concepts are relevant to all forms of research, different criteria are often needed to make these judgements in relation to different research paradigms. However, critical appraisal is based on the idea of **rigour**, which involves a judgement as to whether the research is of a high quality and whether measures were in place to ensure that the research was conducted in an appropriate way, consistent with the underpinning principles associated with the research paradigm.

Polit and Beck (2018) have noted the frequent 'grey areas' in relation to some aspects of research, with experts having different opinions as to what they believe to be appropriate when conducting a study. As research methodologies develop and studies progress, researchers have to weigh up the differing opinions and issues relating to their area of interest and then make decisions about how to proceed with the research. This then has an impact on the overall research outcomes.

In addition, there are often compromises to be made in terms of what is considered ideal and what is practicable in the given situation. These compromises are often related to issues such as sample size, the methods used to collect and analyse data and/or the interpretation of findings. When critically appraising work these decisions can be evaluated by asking questions such as, 'Would another approach have been better?', 'Does the form of analysis have implications for the findings?' or 'Was the sample size sufficient to justify their conclusions?' Decisions can then be made about the quality of the study as a whole and its relevance to clinical practice.

KEY AREAS TO EXPLORE WHEN CRITIQUING A RESEARCH PAPER

Published research papers do tend to have a specific form, being organised into particular sections. Each of these sections is critically examined and certain aspects of each section are considered. The format of papers may vary slightly from journal to journal or appear in a different order when certain research approaches are used. Generally, the content remains the same, with all the aspects appearing in some form. Regardless of the type of research there are several key areas that we should explore and ask questions of when critiquing a research paper. These are:

- The research question
- Literature review (explanation and justification for the study)
- Research design
- Data collection
- Sample
- Data analysis
- Findings
- Discussion
- Applicability to practice (conclusion and recommendations)
- Ethics

The researchers should clearly demonstrate a need for the research (justification) and the question or gap in the knowledge the research sought to address. Research should be conducted not purely for academic attainment but to add to what is already known of the topic. In reading the research paper it should be clear how the reported research builds on previous research. This is often presented in the form of a literature review ending with a clearly articulated research question.

Literature Review

In most published studies, a review of contextual literature is usually present. It should be up to date, and relevant to the research question/hypothesis and proposed objective/aims. Parahoo (2014) suggests four criteria by which to judge a literature review:

1. Whether it provides a rationale for the study. The review should identify why it is important the study is undertaken, the benefits and possible outcomes.
2. Whether it puts the current study into context. It should consider what is already known about the concepts under consideration and provide a balanced view of the various debates around the chosen focus.
3. Whether it provides a review of research relevant to the topic. Research previously conducted should be considered and conclusions drawn, and implications for the proposed study identified.
4. Whether it provides a conceptual/theoretical framework for the research. As you will see below, not all research identifies a theoretical and conceptual framework; however, a literature review should provide an overview of the different frameworks available.

RESEARCH DESIGN

Depending on the question asked will govern the type of research approach used. The research design is the overall plan for the research and should be coherent and appropriate to answer the research question under investigation. Whatever approach is adopted for the study should be the one that best answers the research question. It is for the researchers to explain how they went about conducting the study and why they adopted the approach they did.

The purpose of research is to generate new knowledge, which involves the testing, adjusting and developing of theories. Therefore, there is a need to identify what theory underpins or guides the research process and the design of the study. The terms theoretical framework and conceptual framework are often used interchangeably, although there are distinctions between them – the former usually refers to the use of one theory whereas the latter generally involves the combining of concepts from a range of theories.

Due consideration should also be given to the role of the users' voice in the design of the study. Just as there is increasing emphasis on the need to ensure the user's voice is heard in the organisation and delivery of care, so too has user involvement become central to the research process, not simply as **participants** but rather as part of the whole process. Indeed, in the UK, the Health Research Authority (HRA) has set out its commitment that 'patients, service users and the public are given, and take, the opportunity to participate in health and social care research and to get involved in its design, management, conduct and dissemination, and are confident about doing so' (HRA, 2018: 4).

Activity 5.1

In 2019 the UK Public Involvement Standards Development Partnership issued the UK Standards *for* Public Involvement. This document illustrates the many ways in which users can be involved in research, particularly in the design and implementation of studies. Take the time to read the document using the following link: www.invo.org.uk/wp-content/uploads/2019/11/UK-standards-for-public-involvement-v6.pdf

DATA COLLECTION, ANALYSIS AND RESULTS

These areas relate to the type of information that has been collected, and how it was gathered, processed, analysed and reported. If we think about what factors might affect the quality of the data collected, then we can start to identify the positives and the negatives to those factors that we should look for in a paper. These areas will be explored in greater depth in the following chapters.

In undertaking research, there are many methods that can be used to find answers to questions. Some are more suitable than others. In answering certain types of question, one particular method may be very powerful, but the same method might be weak in dealing with other types of question. Therefore, the relevance of the methods used in the research will be judged in terms of their appropriateness to the nature of the question being asked. Similarly, the sensitivity of the methods must match the needs of the research question.

SAMPLE

The term sampling describes the process used to identify the segment of the population invited to take part in the study. People who form the sample within quantitative research are generally termed **subjects** or **sampling units**. It is important to look at exactly who data were collected from, regardless of the study deign. How important this is will depend on the research question being addressed by the study and the claims it makes about the data. Were the data collected from the subjects of the research question (for example, patients with a particular condition)? Or were they collected from proxies of some sort? – this is often someone representing them, most often a family member, informal carer, or some-times a health professional. Generally, the word **participant** is used in relation to those who take part in qualitative research. This reflects the basic philosophy that individuals take an active role in the research process, rather than being passive subjects.

Researchers identify the target population they are interested in, and this should be specifically described. It could be people with a learning disability who have a particular challenging behaviour or children between the ages of 10 and 16 years who have appen-dicitis. It refers to the entire group; however, data are not usually collected from the entire population, rather a sample is selected.

Look at any characteristics of the sample that are provided (for example, their age, their sex, or level of education) and compare these to the same characteristics of samples in other papers published in the topic area, or, more importantly, to the characteristics of patients in your setting. When considering the sample, it is also worth considering what the response rates were like. How many people were eligible for the study and how many actually took part? Might the people who didn't take part, but were eligible, be different in some way? Might they have given different answers?

Consideration should also be given to the setting that people were drawn from. Were they from primary care, secondary, or some form of specialist care such as a nursing home or hospice? Think about how patients from these settings differ. For example, are patients, with the same diagnosis, but who are in primary care, different in any way to those who might be recruited only from secondary care? How important is it that the sample is population-based?

What setting is of clinical interest to the research question? Which country was it collected from? Different countries have different health systems, which have varying levels of development and funding systems, which may impact on findings.

Different ways of identifying the sample are used in qualitative and quantitative research and are discussed in more detail in Chapters 6 and 7.

Findings and Discussion

Findings are what the researchers found; the discussion is what sense the researchers made of what they found. Polit and Beck (2018) have argued that the discussion should address the main findings of the study and what they mean, consider evidence to support the validity of the findings and examine what limitations may impact on this validity. There is also a need to consider the findings with what is already known about the topic under investigation.

Applicability to Practice

Finally, applicability relates to whether research findings can be implemented in a particular practice setting and these will be highlighted by the researchers in the conclusion and recommendations of a study. To judge applicability, sufficient information must be present within the evidence to identify whether the population sampled in the study is comparable with the population identified in the clinical literature review question. Information related to age, cultural beliefs and values, ethnicity and lifestyle is essential if a judgement is to be made. As with any form of research, while there may be evidence that a particular treatment is effective, there is still a need to consider it in light of specific patient preferences.

Conclusions should ensure that recommendations stated are suitable for the results attained within the capacity of the study. The authors should also concentrate on the limitations in the study and their effects on the outcomes and the proposed suggestions for future studies. Good questions to ask in relation to the conclusions and recommendations include:

- Are the questions posed in the study adequately addressed?
- Are the conclusions justified by the data?
- Do the authors extrapolate beyond the data?
- Are shortcomings of the study addressed and constructive suggestions given for future research?
- Is the conclusion convincing?

Parahoo (2014) suggests that the overarching issues of sources of bias and omissions/exaggeration also need to be considered. Bias is a distortion of the results and/or conclusions and can be introduced in a number of ways – from the participants, the researcher(s), methods of data collection, the environment and the phenomena under study. These will be considered in more depth in relation to qualitative and quantitative approaches in the following chapters.

Ethical Issues

All health service research undertaken in UK care organisations has required formal ethical approval since the Research Governance Framework became law in 2004. Since then, the HRA and the Devolved UK Administrations developed a new UK Policy Framework for Health and Social Care Research which sets out the high-level principles of good practice in the management and conduct of health and social care research in the UK, as well as the responsibilities that underpin high-quality ethical research (HRA, 2018). The regulations governing other countries may vary but the underlying principles are generally the same, reflecting the World Medical Association's (2004) *Declaration of Helsinki* concerning the ethical principles health professionals should consider (see www.wma.net/policies-post/wma-declaration-of-helsinki-ethical-principles-for-medical-research-involving-human-subjects/). Although not legally binding, the declaration has been a major influence on the development of legislation relating to research ethics across the world.

CRITICAL APPRAISAL TOOLS

There are a number of critiquing tools that can help us to make a judgement as to the worth of a research study. Critical appraisal is essentially the assessment of the usefulness of evidence – that means its quality and its applicability to context. We can do this informally, using our knowledge and our personal judgement, taking a common-sense approach to reading a paper or by using informal and formal checklists.

Greenhalgh (2014) has suggested beginning the actual appraisal process by 'getting your bearings' and asking three broad questions:

1. What clinical question is being answered?
2. What type of study is it?
3. Is the design appropriate to the area of research?

By asking these questions decisions can be taken as to whether or not to continue with the appraisal of a particular piece of evidence. If the evidence does not address a question of interest, there is no point in continuing. Identifying the type of study helps with locating an appropriate tool for critique of the work. The appropriateness of the approach is essential in answering clinical questions. If the area of interest is the effectiveness of an intervention but the approach used is one more suitable to considering the feasibility of using a particular intervention then, once again, there is no point in appraising the study. If the study meets all three of these criteria, then the next step is to undertake a full appraisal.

A similar approach known as 'Rapid Critical Appraisal' is put forward by Fineout-Overholt et al. (2010). Here it is suggested that the following key areas are considered:

1. Type of study and place within a hierarchy of evidence.
2. How well it was conducted.
3. Applicability to practice.

Only if a paper meets the criteria related to appropriate levels of evidence, valid results and apparent applicability to practice is it taken forward for full critical appraisal. Appraising the worth of research requires a standardised approach; however, the first decision to be made by any busy clinician is whether to read on. Busy clinicians need to determine quickly which evidence is worth keeping and reading more fully and which can be discarded or is not applicable to their practice.

We see elements of the above two frameworks in the one offered by Polit and Beck (2018), which identifies the broad areas that should be considered in critical appraisal and are relevant to all forms of research (see Table 5.1).

Table 5.1   Elements for critique

Dimension	Issues to be considered
Substantive/ theoretical	Is this an important area to study?
	Does it have relevance to practice?
	Does it take knowledge in this area forward?
	Does the research approach fit with the question to be answered?
Methodological	Are the research design, sampling method, data collection tool and forms of analysis rigorous and appropriate to the research question/ hypothesis?
Practical	Is the scope of the proposed research too broad?
	Have practical issues related to the actual 'doing' of the research been given consideration?
Ethical	Has the researcher identified the ethical issues associated with the research?
	Has ethical approval been sought and given?
Interpretive	Is the researcher's interpretation of the findings credible in light of the data?
	Does the researcher's interpretation appear logical when compared with your own understanding of the area and other research on the topic?
Presentation/style	Is there enough information?
	Is it presented in a clear and concise way?
	Are the themes and arguments developed in a logical and reasoned way?

In addition, Guyatt, Sackett and Cook (1994) suggested that there are three essential questions to be asked when dealing with research involving a therapeutic intervention, as follows:

1. Are the results valid? Do the findings of this study represent the truth? That is, do the results provide an unbiased estimate of the treatment effect, or have they been clouded by bias leading to false conclusions?
2. How precise are the results? If the results are unbiased, they need further examination in terms of precision. The precision would be better in larger studies compared with smaller studies.

3. Are the results applicable to my patient? What are the patient populations, disease and treatments (including comparators) under investigation? What are the benefits and risks associated with the treatment? Do the benefits outweigh the harms?

If the study is an intervention study, what was the intervention? Does the paper tell you enough about it for you to understand what it consisted of? And is the intervention targeting the right thing? Who designed it? And what was the design based on? What evidence was its design based on? Or what theory? Was it relevant evidence or the appropriate theory?

When considering the intervention, it is important to ask who delivered it. What was their skillset and how does that impact on the intervention, or your, or your team's ability to deliver the intervention? As important a question, did those intervention providers have a role in collecting any of the data?

And what did they actually deliver? The intervention may have been well described in the paper, but is there any evidence provided on what was actually delivered? Were the intervention providers faithful to the intervention design? Or did they go a bit off piste? This is known as intervention, or implementation, fidelity.

And if the study was randomised, what was the intervention compared to? What was the 'control condition'? Was it the right control? If it was 'standard' or 'usual care', do you know what 'standard care' means in the context of the study (or country or setting of the study)?

> The following is an example of an informal checklist; it enables you to make a quick assessment of a paper and decide if a greater analysis of the research is warranted. Known as the CRAAP Test it was developed by the librarians at Western University, Canada. As well as having an amusing acronym it focuses on evaluating the quality of information contained in a paper and includes criteria for assessing web-based information. Like a lot of frameworks, it contains a list of questions to help you evaluate the information that you found.
>
> Find a paper on a topic of interest to you and critique it using the CRAAP Test (see Table 5.2). How useful did you find it?

Activity 5.2

Table 5.2   The CRAAP Test critical appraisal tool

The CRAAP Test
Currency: The timeliness of the information.

- When was the information published or posted?
- Has the information been revised or updated?
- Does your topic require current information, or will older sources work as well?
- Are the links functional?

(Continued)

Table 5.2   (Continued)

Relevance: The importance of the information for your needs.

- Does the information relate to your topic or answer your question?
- Who is the intended audience?
- Is the information at an appropriate level (i.e. not too elementary or advanced for your needs)?
- Have you looked at a variety of sources before determining this is one you will use?
- Would you be comfortable citing this source in your research paper?

Authority: The source of the information.

- Who is the author/publisher/source/sponsor?
- What are the author's credentials or organisational affiliations?
- Is the author qualified to write on the topic?
- Is there contact information, such as a publisher or email address?
- Does the URL reveal anything about the author or source? examples: .com .edu .gov .org .net

Accuracy: The reliability, truthfulness and correctness of the content.

- Where does the information come from?
- Is the information supported by evidence?
- Has the information been reviewed or refereed?
- Can you verify any of the information in another source or from personal knowledge?
- Does the language or tone seem unbiased and free of emotion?
- Are there spelling, grammar or typographical errors?

Purpose: The reason the information exists.

- What is the purpose of the information?
- Is it to inform, teach, sell, entertain or persuade?
- Do the authors/sponsors make their intentions or purpose clear?
- Is the information fact, opinion or propaganda?
- Does the point of view appear objective and impartial?
- Are there political, ideological, cultural, religious, institutional or personal biases?

For more information on the framework use the following link: https://researchguides.ben. edu/source-evaluation

Remember, the first thing to consider when reading any research is whether the evidence is from a credible source. If it comes from a journal there are generally some checks already in place – most journals will identify whether or not they subject submissions to peer review. Internet sources do not always have such checks in place; for example, self-publishing sites such as Wikis may have little or no control over the information placed on the web page or its trustworthiness. Decisions will need to be taken as to whether the site is credible – checking an organisation's credentials or asking others what they know about certain sites are useful activities.

FORMAL CRITIQUING TOOLS

A number of tools are available to download free of charge and Table 5.3 details those available from two key organisations, the Critical Appraisal Skills Programme (CASP) and the Joanna Briggs Institute (JBI). All tools have the common aim of aiding in the process of assessing the quality of published literature.

Although qualitative and quantitative approaches are fundamentally different, they do have some common areas for consideration, and these are discussed below. Appendix 3 provides a tool containing general criteria to consider when critiquing an article in this way.

Table 5.3 Example of critical appraisal tools

Published by the Critical Appraisal Skills Programme (CASP) (available at: https://casp-uk.net/casp-tools-checklists/)	Published by the Joanna Briggs Institute (JBI) (available at: https://jbi.global/critical-appraisal-tools)
CASP tools are currently available for the critical appraisal of:	JBI tools are currently available for the critical appraisal of:
<ul><li>Systematic reviews</li><li>Qualitative studies</li><li>Randomised controlled trials</li><li>Case control studies</li><li>Cohort studies</li><li>Clinical prediction rules</li><li>Diagnostic test studies</li><li>Economic evaluations</li></ul>	<ul><li>Systematic reviews</li><li>Qualitative studies</li><li>Randomised controlled trials</li><li>Case control studies</li><li>Cohort studies</li><li>Case reports</li><li>Case series</li><li>Diagnostic test accuracy studies</li><li>Economic evaluations</li><li>Prevalence studies</li><li>Quasi-experimental studies (non-randomised experimental studies)</li><li>Text and opinion</li><li>Analytical cross-sectional studies</li></ul>

Activity 5.3

Using the same paper as you did for Activity 5.2, visit both the CASP and Joanna Briggs sites and find the critiquing tool that best matches your paper's research design. For instance, if a qualitative paper, then use the qualitative critiquing tool from each site. How useful were each of the tools in helping you understand the paper and make a judgement as to its worth? Do you have a preference?

Activity 5.4

Additionally, the Centre for Evidence-Based Medicine has published a range of tools and other resources for the critical appraisal of different types of medical evidence, including clinical trials. Example appraisal sheets are provided together with examples of how to apply them (see www.cebm.ox.ac.uk/resources/ebm-tools/critical-appraisal-tools). Take the time to visit the site and explore their range of critiquing tools, particularly the ones on Prognosis and Diagnostics studies.

CRITIQUING MIXED METHODS RESEARCH

Mixed methods research focuses on collecting, analysing, and mixing both quantitative and qualitative data in a single study or series of studies. Its central premise is that the use of quantitative and qualitative approaches, in combination, provides a better understanding of research problems than either approach alone (Azorin and Cameron, 2010). The purpose of the research remains the same: it should be purposeful and serve an end, by either contributing to the discipline, informing policy or addressing an issue or problem.

Both quantitative and qualitative research have weaknesses. Quantitative research is weak in understanding the context or setting in which data are collected. Qualitative research may include biases and does not lend itself to statistical analysis and generalisation. Mixed method strategies can offset these weaknesses by allowing for both exploration and analysis in the same study. Researchers are able to use all the tools available to them and collect more comprehensive data. This provides results that have a broader perspective of the overall issue or research problem. The final results may include both observations and statistical analyses. Therefore, the results are validated within the study. Using both approaches in one study provides additional evidence and support for the findings.

Mixed methods must comply with the stages of research like any other form of research. A mixed method approach is considered as having been adopted where the mixing of methods occurs within paradigms, sampling, data collection or analytic techniques. The strength of such an approach is that the same issue can be explored from different and consequently fuller perspectives offering a greater understanding of the phenomena under investigation. Mixed methods research tends to be used when one data resource may not be enough to answer the question under investigation; initial results need to be further explained to a greater depth for the study to be of value; when a second method is needed to enhance a primary method, when the project has multi-phases. Multi-method designs are generally intended to supplement one information source with another, or '**triangulate**' on an issue by using different data sources to approach a research problem from different points of view. Greene (2007) identified five purposes of mixing methods (see Table 5.4).

Table 5.4   Greene's five purposes of mixing methods

1. **Triangulation**	Where different methods are used to measure the same phenomenon, to increase confidence in conclusions reached - if consistent or convergent conclusions are reached
2. Complementarity	Where methods are used to investigate different aspects or dimensions of the same phenomena to deepen or broaden the interpretations and conclusions from a study
3. Development	Where results from one method are used to inform the development of other method, e.g. instrument development, but also sampling and implementation
4. Initiation	Where different methods are use to investigate different aspects or dimensions of the same phenomena but, in contrast to complementarity, the intention is divergence in order to generate new understandings
5. Expansion	Where different methods are used to assess different phenomena to expand the scope and range of study

When critiquing mixed methods research, the important thing is to look at how the study combined the methods and how this was able to answer the question rather than using one method or approach. The most common approach to mixing methods is what is known as a Convergent Design. The purpose of this design is 'to obtain different but complementary data on the same topic' (Morse, 1991: 122) to best understand the research problem. The researcher attempts to merge the two data sets, typically by bringing the separate results together in the interpretation or by transforming data to facilitate integrating the two data types during the analysis. For instance, you might collect information by using each method concurrently (at the same time), or sequentially if your aim is to use one method to inform another (say, interviewing before surveying). These two approaches are different. The first is more like two parallel studies that only come together once the data are being analysed, whereas, in the second, the aim is to use the methods in a more integrated way. The actual methods used may be the same, but the ways in which they are sequenced and combined can make a big difference in the process of conducting the study and in the results. As with any research, it is for the researcher(s) to defend and explain their chosen methodology and explain how the research was designed and carried out. When critiquing mixed methods there is a need to consider three factors: the timing of the use of collected data (i.e. the order in which the data are used in a study), the relative weight of the quantitative and qualitative approaches (i.e. the emphasis given to each), and the approach to mixing the two data sets (i.e. how the two data sets will be related or connected).

You will have noticed that neither the CASP nor Joanna Briggs sites above had a mixed methods critiquing tool. This, in part, owes itself to the complexity of mixed methods research. However, there are a number of critiquing tools that specifically look at mixed methods research. The Mixed Methods Appraisal Tool (MMAT) is one such tool, and probably the most well-known.

The MMAT is a critical appraisal tool developed to appraise the methodological quality of empirical studies. Its latest version (version 2018) includes a total of 25 criteria and two screening questions. The MMAT can appraise five different categories of study designs: (a) qualitative, (b) randomised controlled trial, (c) non-randomised, (d) quantitative descriptive and (e) mixed methods studies.

Locate a mixed methods research paper from your field of interest. Have a go at critiquing the paper using the MMAT critiquing tool: http://mixed methodsappraisaltoolpublic.pbworks.com/w/file/fetch/127916259/MMAT_ 2018_criteria-manual_2018-08-01_ENG.pdf

Pay particular attention to how the researcher(s) justified their use of study design in answering the research question. What were the challenges associated with this design? Did the use of mixed methods enhance your understanding of the topic as it was presented within the paper?

Activity 5.5

CRITIQUING CLINICAL GUIDELINES

Clinical guidelines are documents which aim to guide decisions and criteria regarding diagnosis, management and treatment in specific areas of healthcare and are now readily available on a wide range of topics. In the UK, clinical practice guidelines are published primarily by the National Institute for Health and Care Excellence (NICE; www.nice. org.uk/). They are based on the best available evidence and include recommendations by experts, people using services, carers and the public. NICE has published a very useful document outlining the details of the transparency and inclusiveness of the process for the development of UK clinical guidelines (NICE, 2014). Clinical guidelines have become an important aspect of clinical governance as they promote clinical and cost effectiveness and provide a bridge between research and practice.

Sanderlin and Abdul Rahhim (2007) have offered guidance for critiquing clinical practice guidelines, suggesting that while these are important tools in promoting EBP there are various issues to be considered before implementing them. These relate to:

- strength of evidence;
- objective approach to development of guidelines;
- homogeneity of studies – based on studies that have similar designs and complementary results;
- whether study subjects are significantly similar to the relevant patient group;
- whether the guidelines are based on evidence that has been appropriately appraised.

While clinical guidelines are a useful aid to increasing the use of research in the delivery and management of care, they are not without problems, and this has been recognised for some time. For instance, difficulties can be had with regard to the terminology used across sites and clinical practices, difference in clinical settings, lack of a common evidence base, to name but a few. This lack of common ground highlights the need to give careful consideration to guidelines before using them in practice. In an effort to address these issues, processes for guideline development are being generated to ensure that they are produced in a rigorous and appropriate manner.

Many organisations now request that in compiling clinical guidelines developers use the Grades of Recommendation, Assessment, Development and Evaluation (GRADE) process (see www.gradeworkinggroup.org/). This approach provides guidance on how to rate the quality of evidence and strength of recommendations. It provides a 'systematic and transparent framework' for developing guidelines (Guyatt et al., 2011: 380). Guidelines produced using the GRADE approach indicate whether recommendations are based on strong or weak evidence and, therefore, give an indication of the merits of the evidence used. It may be helpful when critically appraising guidelines to identify whether or not the GRADE approach has been used.

The Appraisal of Guidelines Research and Evaluation Collaboration, now the AGREE Research Trust (www.agreetrust.org), provides a tool for appraising clinical guidelines. This international collaboration's aim is to improve the quality and effectiveness of guidelines by promoting a common approach to their development and assessment. The AGREE tool was updated and AGREE II launched in 2009, consisting of 23 criteria organised in six domains. The AGREE Research Trust proposes that the instrument can be used to assess all forms of guidelines (local, national, international) with the exception of quality guidance related to healthcare organisation issues and provides a user's manual to help people with the process of appraisal.

Activity 5.6

Identify a set of guidelines you recently used in practice. Consider these against the AGREE II criteria at www.agreetrust.org. Consider whether or not the guidelines meet the AGREE II criteria.

SKILLS FOR CRITIQUING A PAPER

In developing the skills associated with critical appraisal it is important to remember that to become proficient takes time and that no one is expected to know everything or get it completely right the first time. It is important to know how to find the information needed to conduct the appraisal and to discuss findings with others and ask for their opinions.

To critically appraise evidence a step-by-step approach, as outlined below, will need to be followed, but as confidence and skills grow practitioners also tend to develop their own systems.

1. Identify a suitable checklist to use to critically appraise the evidence.
2. Find somewhere quiet, where you are unlikely to be interrupted.
3. Read through the paper once, so you have a grasp of the content.
4. Read through it again in more depth, evaluating each part of the paper.
5. Make notes or highlight important bits of the paper as you go along.
6. Have a research book to hand so you can check out information or fill in any gaps in your knowledge as you read.
7. Complete the appraisal and discuss your findings with others.

Activity 5.7

The British Medical Journal has collated a list of resources aimed at supporting health professionals to read research papers through a critical lens. Take some time to explore the link below and familiarise yourself with key tips pertaining to each of the difference types of research study.

www.bmj.com/about-bmj/resources-readers/publications/how-read-paper

Summary

- Critical appraisal is associated with published research literature, but there is a need to appraise all forms of evidence.
- Critical appraisal should be an objective consideration of the merits and limitations of the evidence.
- Not all published work is of an appropriate standard or applicable to the practice setting, therefore critical appraisal is a key aspect of EBP.
- Skills of critical appraisal take time to develop and practice is essential.

FURTHER READING

Polit, D.F. and Beck, C.T. (2018) *Essentials of Nursing Research: Appraising Evidence for Nursing Practice* (9th edn). Philadelphia: Lippincott, Williams & Wilkins.

USEFUL WEBLINKS

Critical Appraisal Skills Programme: provides a range of resources to help with developing the skills associated with EBP. It also provides a range of critical appraisal tools. www.casp-uk.net

The Health Research Authority (HRA) is a body of the Department of Health in the UK, set up to protect and promote the interests of patients and the public in health and social care research. It has published or made available a number of key resources about good research practice. See: https://www.hra.nhs.uk/planning-and-improving-research/policies-standards-legislation/

The Joanna Briggs Institute (JBI) is an international not-for-profit, research and development centre within the Faculty of Health and Medical Sciences at the University of Adelaide, South Australia, which provides a wide range of resources to support researchers including a range of tools to aid critical appraisal. http://joannabriggs.org/research/critical-appraisal-tools.html

The National Institute for Health and Care Excellence (NICE) provides national guidance on preventing and treating illness and promoting health. www.nice.org.uk. Specifically in relation to the development of Clinical Guidelines, see: www.nice.org.uk/about/what-we-do/our-programmes/nice-guidance/nice-guidelines/how-we-develop-nice-guidelines

The Royal College of Nursing in the UK provides useful links to resources to aid and inform critical appraisal of evidence. www.rcn.org.uk/library/subject-guides. Specifically: www.rcn.org.uk/library/subject-guides/critical-appraisal and www.rcn.org.uk/library/subject-guides/doing-your-dissertation

6

Critical Appraisal and Quantitative Research

Ros Kane and David Nelson

Learning Outcomes

By the end of the chapter, you will be able to:

- provide an overview of quantitative research approaches;
- identify the key areas for consideration when critically appraising quantitative literature;
- discuss different sampling strategies and methods of analysis used in quantitative research;
- debate issues of reliability and validity.

INTRODUCTION

Research methods refer to the strategies or approaches to the collection and analysis of data and evidence with a view to answering research questions or improving our understanding of a particular topic. Broadly speaking, research methods that are commonly used in healthcare can be categorised overall into either quantitative or qualitative approaches. Researchers are also increasingly using mixed methods where they collect, combine and analyse both quantitative and qualitative data to answer their research questions. Quantitative research is primarily concerned with examining how different **variables** interact and impact on each other. Mantzoukas (2008) found that 51% of research studies published in the top 10 generic nursing journals (such as the *Journal of Advanced Nursing* and the *Journal of Clinical Nursing*) were quantitative in nature. Thus, it is crucial that nurses and other healthcare professionals have a solid understanding of the principles of quantitative research and how to interpret findings from a range of different types of quantitative study.

This chapter briefly outlines some methods used in quantitative research and discusses the issues to be considered when critically appraising quantitative literature. However, it is not intended to provide a full overview of quantitative research, and for a more in-depth exploration you will need to consider some of the recommended reading at the end of the chapter.

WHAT IS QUANTITATIVE RESEARCH?

As identified in Chapter 2, quantitative research has its roots in positivism and in using a deductive approach, starting with a theoretical framework or conceptual model, which predicts how things (variables) behave in the world. Specific predictions (hypotheses) are then deduced from the theory and tested (Polit and Beck, 2018). The aim of quantitative research is, therefore, to explore the relationships between variables and to test hypotheses. It uses objective, rigorous and systematic approaches. A researcher will identify the variables of interest, clearly define what these are and then collect data usually in a numerical form.

A variable, simply put, is something that varies from one person/situation to another. So weight, temperature, pain and personality traits are all variables. Quantitative research seeks to understand why these variations occur. For example, high blood pressure is a variable as not everyone experiences it. If a variable is extremely varied within a particular group it is said to be heterogeneous and where there is limited variability it is described as being homogeneous. Table 6.1 outlines some different types of variables.

Table 6.1   Types of variable

Type	Description
Dependent	The focus of the research (the study is usually conducted to understand the influences on the dependent variable)
	The factor/characteristic or behaviour that the researcher is attempting to understand, describe or affect
Independent	The factor/characteristic or behaviour that is considered to have an influence on the dependent variable
Confounding	A variable that correlates with both the dependent and independent variable. A significant association between the dependent and independent variable may be occurring simply because of the two variables being associated with the confounding variable (also known as a confounding factor or confounder).

Usually, in a quantitative study, the focus is on examining the relationship between independent and dependent variables. For example, you could consider whether age (independent variable) has any implications for the onset of high blood pressure (dependent variable). Whether a variable is identified as dependent or independent depends on the focus of the study. In the above example high blood pressure is the dependent variable, and age is the independent variable. A further study could be conducted to investigate whether there is an association between high blood pressure and other health outcomes such as incidence of coronary artery disease. In this case, high blood pressure would be the independent variable and occurrence of coronary artery disease the dependent variable.

Polit and Beck (2018) suggest quantitative research generally considers specific questions about the relationships, such as:

- the relationship between variables – e.g. is body weight related to the onset of type 2 diabetes?
- the direction of a relationship between variables – e.g. is someone who is overweight more or less likely to develop type 2 diabetes?
- the strength of the relationship between variables – e.g. how likely is it that someone who is overweight will develop type 2 diabetes?
- the cause and effect relationship between the variables – e.g. does being overweight cause the development of type 2 diabetes?

A key element of quantitative research is to determine whether any noted association between two variables is actually a causative association or one that has simply occurred by chance.

Usually, a hypothesis is generated providing a simple statement of the variables to be considered and the relationship between them. For example, I could hypothesise that providing play activities (independent variable) for children prior to surgery will reduce their anxiety (dependent variable). A study could then be designed and conducted to test this hypothesis.

Consider an issue that is causing concern in your area of practice. Identify the variables that might be considered in a study and generate a hypothesis as to the relationship between them.

Activity 6.1

Sample size is an important consideration in quantitative studies. Put simply, the larger the sample, the more power a study has to detect associations which are statistically significant. For more in-depth reading about sample size calculations please refer to the recommended reading at the end of the chapter. Usually, a large number of people are recruited into quantitative research studies, and statistical tests are used to analyse the data and enable these to be presented in a succinct form. Statistics also help in making judgements regarding the level of statistical significance of research findings.

Analysis is an attempt to measure the concepts and variables under consideration as accurately and objectively as possible. Objectivity is seen as a central tenet of quantitative research, with the researcher viewed as 'standing outside' the research process. The intention here is to ensure that neither the researcher nor the subjects introduce any form of bias into the research process. Bias is where the results of a study are distorted for some reason (this, along with ways to reduce bias, will be considered in more detail later in the chapter). To reduce bias a process known as blinding is often used. Here, information relating to the research process is concealed from those on whom the research is conducted and/or those involved in delivering the intervention being studied. For example, if the effectiveness of a particular drug is being tested, an experimental group of subjects receive the drug and a control group receive a placebo. The subjects and/or those administering the drug may not be made aware of who is receiving it and who is receiving the placebo. If information is withheld from only one of the groups involved – the subjects or those administering the drug – it is called a single-blind study. If information is withheld from both groups it would be known as a double-blind study.

TYPES OF QUANTITATIVE RESEARCH

Generally, two types of research design are present within quantitative research: experimental and non-experimental.

Experimental approaches, such as randomised control trials (RCTs), actively introduce a treatment or intervention in an attempt to study causal relationships. The aim is to identify whether a particular intervention has an impact on the dependent variable. To be a true experimental design the following three conditions must be met:

1. An intervention is controlled by a researcher so some subjects receive the intervention and others do not.
2. At least two groups of subjects are involved – a control group and an experimental group.
3. Random selection and allocation of subjects to research groups will occur.

If these three conditions are not all met, the research is described as quasi-experimental. Quasi-experimental approaches are used to test the effectiveness of interventions and are often done when it is not possible to meet one of the three conditions above.

Concerns have been raised in relation to the quality of the reporting of experimental studies. It is suggested that frequently the information given is not sufficient to allow proper critical appraisal. To address these concerns, guidelines as to what should be included in reports of RCTs have been generated; these are known as the CONSORT (Consolidated Standards of Reporting Trials) statement (Schulz et al., 2010). Various 'extensions' to the CONSORT statement have been developed to give guidance on specific designs, data and interventions. Statements related to other forms of quantitative research are also being developed. These may be of help in identifying what should be included in quantitative research studies.

Activity 6.2

Visit the CONSORT website at www.consort-statement.org and use the CONSORT statement to identify the aspects that are considered to be central to the design and writing up of randomised control trials (RCTs).

Non-experimental quantitative research is used to describe and/or identify associations between variables and would generally be used to address Polit and Beck's (2018) first three questions (see above). However, it is not possible to definitively establish cause and effect relationships. Instead, the intention is to explore potential associations – possibly with a view to establishing firm causative relationships in future research. Key examples of non-experimental study designs are outlined below.

Cross-sectional studies collect data at a single point in time (for example, by doing a survey of a population). They may also be used to make comparisons between different groups within that population. For example, if you wanted to measure whether the length of time someone was in residential care impacts on their level of satisfaction, you might collect data at the same point from current residents, ask how long they had been in residential care and compare levels of satisfaction between those who had lived in the setting for three months, six months, nine months and twelve months.

Longitudinal studies (also known as cohort studies) collect data at various points over an extended period of time from an identified individual/group of people. For example, if you were interested in the impact of socioeconomic factors on the health outcomes of children from birth to the age of six you would collect data from the same group of children from birth to the age of six years at defined intervals (perhaps at six-month intervals).

Retrospective studies collect data after an event and look back or ask questions relating to historical situations. For example, patients' notes may be examined for information in relation to a specific treatment and recovery. It is possible to make comparisons between two different groups (case control studies), such as those who developed a particular disease and those who remained free from disease.

Prospective studies collect data in relation to a specific independent variable and the dependent variable is measured at a later date. In this approach it would be possible, for example, to consider if coping behaviours in relation to stress have an impact on incidence of myocardial infarctions by measuring stress-coping behaviours in a population and then identifying the number of people who had a myocardial infarction in 10 years' time.

It is important to differentiate between **descriptive** and **correlation studies**. Descriptive studies generally observe, describe and document areas of interest as they occur naturally. Correlation studies examine relationships between variables. Again, as identified in relation to RCTs, reporting guidelines have been created with regard to a number of these approaches and can be found at the EQUATOR network website (www.equator-network.org/).

CRITICAL APPRAISAL

As identified in Chapter 5, there are a number of tools available to help you critically appraise the different types of quantitative research. Therefore, it is important to use the correct checklist to help you focus on the most important aspects of the study. Appendix 3 gives a generic approach to particular areas to be addressed in this form of critique – those specific to quantitative research are highlighted (Appendix 4), and an overview is given below. For discussion of the other general items see Chapter 5. Remember, when doing a critical appraisal it is helpful to have a good research book to hand so information can be clarified along the way.

Activity 6.3

Find a quantitative research study relevant to your area of practice and an appropriate critical appraisal tool.

Hypothesis/research question and research objectives/aims

Not all quantitative research has a hypothesis, particularly descriptive studies. However, there should always be a clearly stated research question. If a hypothesis is required this should be a simple statement identifying the relationship between at least two clearly stated variables and it should be testable. Different types of hypotheses include the following:

- Directional – suggests the nature and direction of the relationship between variables: positive (e.g. increased physical activity improves mental functioning); inverse/negative (e.g. people with learning disabilities display less challenging behaviour when involved in diversional activities); difference (e.g. people with high blood pressure are more likely to suffer from a coronary artery disease than those who do not have high blood pressure).
- Non-directional – this only suggests that a relationship might exist (e.g. children differ from adults in the levels of anxiety they experience on admission to hospital).
- Null hypothesis – where no relationship is suggested (e.g. there is no relationship between the use of cognitive behavioural therapy and an improvement of mood in people who are depressed).

The aims/objectives of the research should also be clearly identified and reflect the research question and/or hypothesis.

Operational definitions

It is expected that concepts used within the research will be defined. For example, if a study related to whether wound dressing X is more effective than wound dressing Y in the treatment of leg ulcers, there is a need to clearly define what is meant by wound dressings X and Y, leg ulcer, the procedures to be used when applying the dressing and the effects to be measured. While words such as 'leg ulcer' are in common usage, within the research context there is a need to identify precisely what type of leg ulcers are to be considered. Without this type of information the rigour and the generalisability of the findings can be called into question and the ability to identify if the research is relevant to a specific area of practice is compromised.

Read the article chosen in the previous activity. Identify the operational definitions and appraise whether these are sufficiently described to allow you to
identify applicability to your own area of practice.

Activity 6.4

Data collection methods

The measurement tools selected to collect data must be appropriate to the research question/
hypothesis and the operational definitions and should also collect the type and level of
data required. Data collection methods in quantitative research can take many forms –
questionnaires, observational schedules, self-reporting schedules or bio-physiological
measures. All of these approaches involve the measurement of variables through the
assignment of numbers to the variable according to pre-agreed rules. For example, there
are identified rules and methods for measuring weight, which allow you to observe what
someone weighs. However, not all variables are easily measured and methods of measurement
have to be agreed to allow measurement to be taken.

In considering measurement in quantitative research there is a need to understand:

* what is being measured;
* how it is being measured;
* why it is being measured in this way;
* what the rules are in relation to that measurement (Parahoo, 2014).

Without this information it is not possible to judge whether the data being collected
are accurate.

There are two main criteria for assessing the research tools – reliability and validity –
which are both discussed in more detail below. However, briefly, reliability of measurement
tools relates to the accuracy with which a tool measures the variable, whether it is able to
reproduce findings consistently and be free from error. Validity relates to whether the tool
measures what it is meant to measure. Frequently, researchers use tools that have already been
tested for reliability and validity. If a new tool is being used then there should be evidence
that it has been pre-tested for its reliability/validity.

Data collection protocols are usually produced by quantitative researchers identifying
procedures for collecting data. Clear instructions as to what conditions should be met
and any specific instruction in relation to the sequencing of collecting and recording of
information are expected to be present.

Sampling

Studies almost always involve samples rather than the whole population of interest. If findings
are to be generalised to the population of interest, then the sample must be representative of
the whole of that population. For example, a seminar group of 30 nursing students where 15

are studying adult nursing and 15 are studying mental health nursing could potentially generate a representative sample that includes 10 students: five studying adult nursing and five mental health nursing. The sample size required for a particular study is often determined through the use of power calculations. Statistical power is the ability of a study to detect statistically significant results. The power of a test is affected by the sample size, and power calculations will identify the sample size needed to detect significant differences where they exist. A well-designed study will identify the use of power calculations in calculating sample sizes.

Quantitative research generally uses what is known as probability sampling. In this type of sample every unit within the population of interest has an equal chance of being selected. To ensure representativeness, random selection procedures are used. Appropriate randomisation is of central importance as it ensures that neither the researchers nor the subjects will be able to influence characteristics of the population under study. Four approaches to probability sampling are available – simple, stratified, cluster and systematic (see Table 6.2).

It is important that clear and precise accounts of the inclusion and exclusion criteria are documented within the study in order that the exact characteristics of the population used for the collection of data are known. Inclusion criteria are characteristics that the

Table 6.2   Types of randomised sampling

Type	Description
Simple random sampling	A sampling frame is generated listing all the elements of the population
	A number is allocated to each one of the elements
	A table of random grouped numbers (computer generated) is used to select sample units for specified sample size
Stratified random sampling	Ensures subgroups (e.g. age, ethnicity) within a population are present in the sample in the same proportions
	Proportional stratified sampling = sample proportions are same as population
	Disproportional sampling = a large sample of a particular subgroup is needed to consider the relationship between variables in that group
	Weighting = adjustments made to statistical analysis to provide actual population values
	Simple random sampling is used to select the subjects from each subgroup
Cluster random (multi-stage) sampling	Used in large-scale studies with a widespread geographical population
	Clusters of target population randomly selected
	Units within each cluster again randomly selected to be part of the sample
	Simple random sampling would be used at each stage
Systematic random sampling	Sample units are selected at predetermined intervals, e.g. every 5th or 7th or 20th unit on sampling frame
	Interval used decided by dividing the available target population by the sample size required, e.g. 100 units for a sample of 20 = every 5th unit selected ($100 \cdot 20 = 5$)
	Sample frame itself is randomised before using this form of sampling

prospective subjects must have if they are to be included in the study, while exclusion criteria are those characteristics that disqualify prospective subjects from inclusion in the study. Without this information, the generalisability of findings to other client groups will be called into question, therefore reducing your ability to make decisions as to the applicability of the research to your own area of practice.

Data analysis

Statistical analysis allows quantitative researchers to make sense of the mass of numbers generated in the collection of data. There are four levels of data within quantitative research – nominal, ordinal, interval and ratio (see Box 6.1). The level of data indicates the statistical test to be used. It is beyond the scope of this chapter to give a full account of all forms of data test and analysis. However, some books are recommended at the end of this chapter.

Zellner et al. (2007) having reviewed over 400 research articles in various nursing journals found that 80% of these used the same 10 statistical approaches (see Box 6.2 for a description of these 10 approaches). Further books on study design and statistical techniques are recommended at the end of this chapter.

Box 6.1   Levels of measurement of variables

- *Nominal* - simply categorises groups (e.g. male or female) and assigns a code number to the identifying traits, for example, Male = 1, Female = 2. Allows the identification of the frequency of a trait within a category - for example, identifying that 60% of a sample were female.
- *Ordinal* - codes information according to an order in relation to specified criteria. Likert scales produce ordinal data (e.g. strongly agree, agree, neither agree nor disagree, disagree, strongly disagree).
- *Interval* - rank ordering of characteristics, in which the distance between any two numbers on the scale is known (e.g. temperature scale).
- *Ratio* - ordering of a trait, the intervals between each rank and the absolute magnitude of the trait (e.g. height or weight).

Box 6.2   Description of statistical tests most commonly used in nursing and health research

Descriptive statistics

- *Mean* - the average sum of a set of values. If the ages of six people were iden- tified as 26, 29, 30, 38, 40 and 41, the mean age would be 34 (26 + 29 + 30 + 38 + 40 + 41 = 204 / 6 = 34).

(Continued)

- *Frequency distribution* – the arrangement of data in ascending order (lowest to highest value), identifying the number of times a particular value or score occurs. If the stress levels of 50 people prior to surgery were measured and given a numerical score (ranging from 1 to 10) it might result in the following frequency distribution:

  o   Frequency 2 3 5 8 11 7 6 4 3 1 (n 50)
  o   Score 1 2 3 4 5 6 7 8 9 10

- *Standard deviation* – the average deviation of the values from the mean.
- *Range* – the distance between highest and lowest values and gives a picture of the dispersion of data (the range between 15% and 85% = 70).
- *Percentages, percentiles and quartiles* – the frequency at which something occurs is reported in percentages, e.g. 60% of people prefer butter to margarine; a percentile is the point below which a specific percentage of values lies (a score at a 60th percentile means 60% of scores are below that); quartiles divide distribution scores into four equal parts.

Inferential statistics

- *t-test* – examines the difference between the means of two sets of values.
- *Analysis of variant* (ANOVA) – examines the difference between several means.
- *Correlation* – identifies an association between variables where a variation in one is related to a variation in another.
- *Cronbach's alpha* – a reliability index used to measure internal consistency of a multi-itemed measurement tool such as an anxiety scale or an assessment tool.
- *Chi-squared* – compares data collected in the form of frequencies or percentages.

Briefly, statistics are identified as being either descriptive or inferential. Descriptive statistics, as the term suggests, 'describe' and summarise the data, often in the form of averages and percentages. Within the EBP movement one of the most useful forms of descriptive statistics in decision making are effect/risk measures. These measures are used to calculate the 'clinical meaningfulness' of findings and are frequently seen in systematic reviews. However, these are also being increasingly included in research reports and it may be useful for you to explore these in more depth.

Inferential statistics allow researchers to make 'inferences' (draw conclusions) about the specific relationships between variables. The type of test used usually depends on:

- the sampling method;
- the level of data required (e.g. nominal);
- the distribution of variables to be measured.

Parametric tests are usually adopted where the sample is randomised, where there is a normal distribution of variables. These types of test are generally seen to be more powerful that non-parametric tests. Non-parametric tests do not consider a particular form of distribution to be present, and can be used with nominal and also ordinal data and on small samples.

Statistical tests that identify significance – whether an observed result is the product of chance or represents a finding of significance – are based on probability theory. This is commonly referred to as a p value, the smaller the p value the less likely the possibility that the result has occurred by chance. It is conventionally expressed as $p < 0.05$, though this cut-off is arbitrary (the symbol $<$ identifies it is less than; $>$ would signify more than). Significance levels of $0.05, 0.01$ and 0.001 are the most commonly cited p values in relation to significance of findings. A value of 0.05 identifies that the results are significant at a 5% level, meaning that there is a less than five chances in a hundred (or 1 in 20) likelihood that the result has occurred by chance. The p value of 0.05 is generally accepted as the level at which it is possible to claim a positive result. There are two commonly used tests to consider significance – chi-squared and t-test:

- The chi-squared test identifies significance between groups.
- The t-test identifies differences between groups.

Where statistical significance is identified, confidence intervals are usually calculated to work out how precise the results are. The wider the interval, the less likely the same results would be found if the research was to be repeated a number of times. If you found that wound dressing X improved wound healing in 65% of the sample, there is a need to know how precise that estimate is if it is to be applied to the wider population. The sample result is unlikely to be exactly the same as the population response to the treatment. It is possible to calculate an interval (with an upper and lower limit) in relation to the sample result that suggests the range within which the target population response to treatment will fall. If the confidence interval had a lower limit of 25% and a higher limit of 100%, the confidence interval is very wide and, therefore, the value of 65% is very imprecise. If, however, the confidence interval is between 60 and 70%, the estimate of 65% is more precise and more meaningful. By convention, researchers usually report confidence intervals of 95% (expressed as 95% CI), which are the range of values (the interval) within which there is 95% confidence that the real value applies to the total population of patients.

Findings

It is usually the norm that descriptive statistics are presented first, to give the readers an overview of the variables. Findings are then generally ordered in terms of importance or in relation to the sequencing of the research question/hypotheses. Tables are used where a number of statistical tests are reported. Tables should be presented in a clear and easily understandable manner, with clear links to the written narrative. All data should be accounted for.

Reliability, validity and applicability

Reliability relates to the accuracy and consistency of findings, whether the same results would be reached if the same variables were repeatedly measured in the same way

(Bowling, 2014). For example, you may be fairly sure that a thermometer will accurately measure your temperature and that it would give the same results on repeated measurement at five-minute intervals. If two results varied by five degrees, the reliability of the thermometer would need to be questioned. In critically appraising research, the reader is assessing whether the research design, methodology and measurement tools provide accurate findings and whether, if repeated, the same results would be found.

Validity is described by Polit and Beck (2018) as a property of inference. Researchers can only infer that a perceived effect is a result of their hypothesised case if the research is valid: namely, that there is confidence that what was intended to be measured has been measured. Four types of validity are proposed by Polit and Beck:

1. Statistical conclusion validity – where tests are deemed to be appropriate/fair and any identified statistical relationship between the variables is based on sound evidence.
2. Internal validity – where a relationship is proven that this is the result of the independent variable, not some other circumstance, such as chance, confounding variables, introduction of bias, etc. (see Table 6.3).
3. Construct validity – relates to the degree a tool measures the thing it is designed to measure. For instance, you may be fairly sure that a thermometer is a valid tool to measure temperature (unless it's broken in some way) but you might be less sure of a tool designed to measure pain.
4. External validity – concerns the generalisability of findings to other people and/or settings.

Table 6.4 gives an overview of some of the issues that threaten validity in relation to the above items.

Table 6.3   Sources of bias

Type	Description
Selection bias	Inadequate randomisation or systematic error in the way participants are recruited into a study
Performance bias	Differences in the way intervention is received/delivered
Attrition bias	More subjects are lost from one research group than another (control or experimental)
Detection bias	Differences which occur when assessing outcomes of RCTs
Participant bias	A lack of full disclosure or giving what is considered to be appropriate responses
Conceptual bias	Faulty conceptualisation of problem, interpretation of findings or drawing of conclusions
Design bias	Faults in any aspect of the research design
Recall bias	Difficulties relating to recalling past events, memory degeneration over time

Validity can also be compromised by confounding variables. As discussed earlier, confounding variables are where a proposed relationship between two variables may actually be due to a third variable. In critically appraising studies you must consider whether the researcher has considered potential confounding variables in the research design and analysis of the findings.

Table 6.4   Factors that may affect validity

Type of validity	Threats to validity
Statistical conclusion	Sample size is small
	Tools lacking the precision to accurately measure the variables
	Variations in the implementation of an intervention
	Treatment adherence
Construct validity	Hawthorne or placebo effect – people's behaviour as a response to being observed or to treatment because they believe it will have a positive effect
	Researcher's response to subjects encourages certain responses
	Novelty effect – perception of new treatments may result in positive or negative responses from subjects
	Compensation – control group subjects are 'compensated' in some way by health staff or family for not receiving research intervention
	Contamination – control and experimental group receive similar services generally or experimental group member moves to control group by dropping out of the trial

Choose and locate a quantitative article of interest and critically appraise it using the questions in Appendix 4. Identify aspects where you need to develop further skills and knowledge. Then develop an action plan outlining how you will develop the knowledge and skills you require to complete the task appropriately.

Activity 6.5

Summary

- The aim of quantitative research is to explore relationships between variables and test hypotheses. The researcher identifies the variables of interest, clearly defines what these are and then collects data, usually in a numerical form.
- The relationships between independent variables and dependent variables are considered. Statistics help in making judgements and generalisations of the value of the research findings for the research population as a whole.

(Continued)

- Two types of research design are present within quantitative research: experimental and non-experimental.
- Quantitative research generally uses what is known as probability sampling.
- There are four levels of measurement within quantitative research – nominal,
  ordinal, interval and ratio. The level of measurement indicates the statistical
  test to be used.

FURTHER READING

Bowling, A. (2014) *Research Methods in Health* (4th edn). New York: Open University Press.

Carneiro, I. (2017) *Introduction to Epidemiology (Understanding Public Health)* (3rd edn). Maidenhead: Open University Press.

Parahoo, K. (2014) *Nursing Research: Principles, Process and Issues* (3rd edn). Basingstoke: Palgrave Macmillan.

Saks, M. and Allsop, J. (2012) *Researching Health: Qualitative, Quantitative and Mixed Methods* (2nd edn). London: Sage.

Scott, I. and Mazhindu, D. (2014) *Statistics for Health Care Professionals: An Introduction* (2nd edn). London: Sage.

USEFUL WEBLINKS

CONSORT website: provides explanations and examples of what is expected to be included in some forms of quantitative research. www.consort-statement.org

Critical Appraisal Skills Programme Checklists: provide a range of checklists to help with critiquing quantitative studies, including tools for systematic reviews, randomised control trials, cohort studies, case control studies, economic evaluations and diagnostic studies. www.casp-uk.net/casp-tools-checklists

Netting the Evidence: an extremely useful online resource, for those involved in and wishing to further their knowledge of evidence based practice. www.nettingtheevidence.org.uk

RCN Critical Appraisal Subject Guide: provides links to a range of key resources in relation to critical appraisal tools and checklists. www.rcn.org.uk/library/subject-guides/critical-appraisal

7

Critical Appraisal and Qualitative Research

Paul Linsley and Janet Barker

Learning Outcomes

By the end of the chapter, you will be able to:

- discuss qualitative research and its basic traits;
- list qualitative forms of data collection;
- identify the key areas for consideration when critically appraising qualitative literature;
- identify criteria used for evaluating the rigour of qualitative studies.

INTRODUCTION

This chapter considers the methods and approaches used in qualitative research and discusses the issues which should be considered when critically appraising literature of this type. However, as with the previous chapter, it is not the intention to provide a full overview of the research process, and for a more in-depth explanation you need to explore some of the recommended reading at the end of the chapter.

There remains a tendency to equate the idea of 'evidence' with quantitative data produced in the context of experimental or well-controlled quasi-experimental research. Indeed, such research continues to provide the foundation on which healthcare policy is built and debated and sits higher in the hierarchy of evidence. This situation is being challenged on a number of fronts and there is a growing recognition of the importance of qualitative research in informing and shaping clinical practice.

WHAT IS QUALITATIVE RESEARCH?

Qualitative research is a broad term for a variety of research approaches and is often seen as being the opposite to and invariably at odds with quantitative research. It has different philosophical underpinnings, which give rise to different ways of thinking about the nature of knowledge and how this can be generated.

Broadly speaking, qualitative research can be defined as 'an iterative process in which improved understanding is achieved by making new significant distinctions resulting from getting closer to the phenomenon studied' (Aspers and Corte, 2019: 139). Whereas positivistic or quantitative research assumes that phenomena are best understood from an objective standpoint, qualitative research assumes that meaning and knowledge are constructed through the eyes of the people that they study (for example, Gregory et al., 2019).

Qualitative research often involves asking participants about their experiences of things that have happened or are happening to them in their lives. It aims to make sense of or interpret phenomena in terms of meanings people bring to them. It provides answers to questions such as, 'what it is to have and live with a particular illness, what does dignity and respect mean to people, why did the person use that service and not another and what might work better for our users' (NHS England, 2017: 2). In doing so, the researcher attempts to understand the person's worldview through a variety of methods and focuses on the interpretation of words, how people describe their experiences, perspectives, understanding beliefs and values. It is suggested that qualitative research has six central traits (see Table 7.1).

Table 7.1   Six basic traits of qualitative research

Trait	Description
Belief in multiple realities	There is no one reality/truth
	People actively construct their understanding of the world
	People have different experiences of life
	A number of perspectives are available in relation to any situation/phenomenon
	Appreciates complexity and multiple realities
An understanding of the nature of the phenomena being studied through appropriate methods is provided	There are multiple ways of understanding various phenomena
	The most appropriate approach(es) to 'capturing' these understandings must be used
	The phenomenon under consideration dictates the method to be used
	Multiple forms of data collection are often used to ensure a full understanding of the research topic
	Conducts analysis along with data collection

Trait	Description
Provides an understanding from the subject/ participant's point of view	Qualitative research involves developing a theory in relation to a phenomenon – asking questions such as 'what do you experience of caring?' from someone with a learning disability
	Generates understanding from patterns
Research is conducted in the natural environment in which the phenomenon occurs	No attempt is made to control the environment
	Focuses on interpreting and understanding a social construction of meaning in a natural setting
	The natural environment provides a way of accessing the participant's perspective whilst in the 'space' that it occurs
	Gives access to any cues or influences on the individual's perspective
The researcher as part of the process	Acceptance that all research is conducted in a subjective way
	Researcher is seen as adding to the richness of the data
Data are said to be 'rich' and 'deep'	Data are collected in the form of words, describing the perspectives and experiences of the participants

(Adapted from Streubert and Carpenter, 2010)

TYPES OF QUALITATIVE RESEARCH

One of the difficulties of critiquing qualitative research is that there are many different approaches to doing it (Moorley and Cathala, 2019). This is because there are many ways to view the lived experience of others, and because different researchers come from different traditions, each with their own theoretical and philosophical underpinnings (Mohajan, 2018). The most common approaches are outlined below, and an overview of their various aspects is presented in Table 7.2. As with quantitative research, the method adopted for a qualitative study must be that which best answers the research question.

Phenomenology

This approach is based in a philosophical tradition developed by Edmund Husserl (1857–1938) and Martin Heidegger (1889–1976), which considers people's everyday experiences. The focus here is to explore the meaning that people attach to their lived experience and is closely related to **hermeneutics**, which centres on meaning and interpretation – how people interpret their experiences within a specific context. For example, if you wanted to know what it means to someone to be given a diagnosis of cancer, how they experience this, you might undertake a phenomenological study.

Key question: What are the meaning, structure and essence of the lived experience of this phenomenon by an individual(s)?

Grounded theory

Developed by sociologists Glaser and Strauss (1967), grounded theory is an approach originally forwarded as a way of developing theories and hypotheses that are 'grounded' in the data collected. Strauss and Corbin (1990: 7) describe a grounded theory as one that 'is discovered, developed, and provisionally verified through systematic data collection and analysis of data pertaining to the phenomenon'. It is based on the idea that human behaviour is developed through people's interactions and their interpretation of these. It is often used to study social processes, considering the changes that occur over time in relation to particular experiences. In nursing it is frequently used to gain an understanding of the process through which people learn to manage and/or adapt to a new situation. For example, this approach could be used to consider how children adapt their lives over time following a diagnosis of diabetes.

Key question: What theory or explanation emerges from an analysis of the data collected about this phenomenon?

Ethnography

This research approach has its roots in anthropology, being used to consider beliefs, values and shared meanings of people in particular cultures. Leininger (1985: 35) defined ethnography as 'the systematic process of observing, detailing, describing, documenting and analysing the lifeways or particular patterns of a culture (or subculture)'. Cultures in this context could relate to an entire social group (such as the culture of people from Romania) or to a small group (such as a particular ward setting). Therefore, you could study the beliefs and values of people from Romania in relation to the care of people with learning disabilities. Alternatively, you could study how the culture of a particular residential home for people with learning disabilities impacts on the care given.

Key question: What are the cultural characteristics of this group of people or this cultural setting?

Action research

Action research can include both qualitative and quantitative approaches and is used to study the effects of actions when these are taken to change or improve something. There are various forms of action research, but the basic tenet is that it is a group activity (Streubert and Carpenter, 2010), usually involving some form of collaboration between the researcher and the participants – practitioners, patients or other stakeholders in the process – with a view to improving/changing practices in a specific area. It is also said to be context bound, in that the research is undertaken because of a defined issue related to a specific area. Its participants are seen as central to decision-making processes and have the final say as to whether changes are implemented or not. It is often seen as cyclic in nature, with problems being identified, changes made and impact evaluated. For instance, this approach could be used to consider the most appropriate way to change how 'clinical handover' is organised in a particular ward setting.

Key question: What have we learnt from implementing this change?

Discourse analysis

Discourse analysis is relatively new to nursing research and looks at the ways in which people talk about particular issues; for example, the systems people use in communicating with each other. It tries to uncover the rules that govern how people talk about things. Its basic premise is that language is not neutral: when talking, what is said and how it is said has particular meaning and intentions. Foucault's (1979) work has been particularly influential in this area, focusing on how power is exercised through the use of language. For example, it would be possible to consider what power relations are present when qualified nurses talk to students and what values are present in the language they use.

Key question: How is the information presented and whose interest does it serve?

Historical research

As a research approach, historical methods collect and interpret historical data in a systematic way. The aim is to provide new insights into a topic area, not to summarise existing knowledge as might be done with a literature review (Streubert and Carpenter, 2010). Generally, the form of historical research is underpinned by a particular theoretical framework, such as feminism or postmodernism. Historical research may be in the form of biographical accounts of individuals who provide oral histories of particular groups; for example, oral histories could be taken from people who have experienced mental health institutions at various points in the twentieth century.

Key question: What can we learn from what has gone before?

Case study

Another popular form of qualitative research is the use of a case study. A case study refers to an in-depth analysis of a single person, a group of people, an organisation or an institution, often as a series of vignettes. Case studies can be quite complex in their design and track a person or series of events over time. According to Yin (2018), a case study design should be considered when: (a) the focus of the study is to answer 'how' and 'why' questions; (b) you cannot manipulate the behaviour of those involved in the study; (c) you want to cover contextual conditions because you believe they are relevant to the phenomenon under study; or (d) the boundaries are not clear between the phenomenon and context.

Key question: What is happening or has happened? How or why did something happen the way it did?

While the relationships between theory and qualitative methods may appear complex, they provide the 'scaffolding' (Anfara and Mertz, 2006) from which researchers go about constructing and conducting their studies. Furthermore, while qualitative researchers will claim to use a particular approach to their study, it is not unusual to see a combining of data collection methods; for example, case study data may be used and analysed using grounded theory. One of the strengths of qualitative research is its responsiveness to a changing situation and its ability to pursue new lines of enquiry as they emerge.

Activity 7.1

Find one piece of research for each of the research approaches identified in Table 7.2 relevant to your own field of practice. Consider how each piece might inform your practice and how it shapes your understanding of the topic under investigation. The example papers we use here all look at different aspects of nursing practice using different qualitative methodology.

Table 7.2   Overview of qualitative research approaches

Approach	Types of research questions	Data collection	Example
Phenomenology	Meaning/lived experience	Unstructured interviews	Arcadi, P., Simonetti, V., Ambrosca, R., Cicolini, G., Simeone, S., Pucciarelli, G., Alvaro, R., Vellone, E. and Durante, A. (2021) 'Nursing during the COVID-19 outbreak: a phenomenological study', *Journal of Nursing Management*, 29(5): 1111–19.
Grounded theory	Social settings Process questions	Interviews Observation	Rooddehghan, Z., ParsaYekta, Z. and Nasrabadi, A.N. (2019) 'Equity in nursing care: a grounded theory study', *Nursing Ethics*, 26(2): 598–610.
Ethnography	Culture Beliefs and values	Participant observation Field notes Interviews	Martin-Ferreres, M.L., De Juan Pardo, M.Á., Bardallo Porras, D. and Medina Moya, J.L. (2019) 'An ethnographic study of human dignity in nursing practice', *Nursing Outlook*, 67(4): 393–403.
Action research	Implementing change	Mixed	Williamson, T., Rawle, A., Bacon, E., et al. (2006) *An Evaluation of a Nurse Led Unit: An Action Research Study*. University of Salford, Manchester: Monograph. https://usir.salford.ac.uk/id/eprint/12868/
Discourse analysis	Verbal interaction What power relationships are present in conversations?	Observation Recording of interactions Field notes	Fejes, A. (2008) 'Governing nursing through reflection: a discourse analysis of reflective practices', *Journal of Advanced Nursing*, 64(3): 243–50.
Historical	Identifying historical roots and/or practices	Interviews Narratives Documentation	Xavier, M.L., Carvalho, M.E.B de, Goncalves, M.B. dos S., et al. (2021) 'The use of photography as a research source on historical studies on nursing', *Research, Society and Development*, 10(5): 1–13.

Approach	Types of research questions	Data collection	Example
Case study	How or why a thing happened the way it did	Analysis of an event presented as a written account or presentation	Shaban, R.Z., Considine, J., Fry, M. and Curtis, K. (2017) 'Case study and case-based research in emergency nursing and care: theoretical foundations and practical application in paramedic pre-hospital clinical judgement and decision-making of patients with mental illness', *Australian Emergency Nursing Journal*, 20: 17–24.

CRITICAL APPRAISAL

As we have seen, qualitative research aims to make sense of, or interpret, phenomena in terms of the meanings people bring to them. Just like quantitative research, qualitative research will address a clinical problem through a clearly formulated question, and just like in quantitative research, the analysis of qualitative data should be done using explicit, systematic, and reproducible methods (Soilemezi and Lincenviciute, 2018).

However, there has been a great deal of debate and disagreement about what the appropriate criteria are for critically appraising qualitative research. As Greenhalgh noted (1997: 243), 'by its very nature, qualitative research is non-standard, unconfined, and dependent on the subjective experience of both the researcher and the researched. It explores what needs to be explored and cuts its cloth accordingly. It is debateable, therefore, whether an all-encompassing critical appraisal checklist … could ever be developed.' Furthermore, there is disagreement on the characteristics defining good qualitative research, and even whether criteria for qualitative research should exist at all (Collins and Stockton, 2018).

Some of this situation owes itself to the very nature of qualitative research. Some of the most important qualities of qualitative research are the hardest to measure. For example, a study may be judged to have followed the appropriate procedures for a particular approach, to have given information on the selection of participants, and provided clear details of the method followed, yet the study may suffer from poor interpretation and offer little insight into the phenomenon at hand.

Contradictions also occur because there is more than one qualitative approach (just like quantitative research). In quantitative research we have both generic and specific critical appraisal tools for each of the different study designs. If we want them there are specific tools for randomised controlled trials, cohort studies and so on. In qualitative research there is also a range of different approaches or theoretical perspectives (e.g. studies might use a grounded theory framework or discourse analysis framework), as well as a range of methods (e.g. interviews, focus groups, observations). So, ideally, we need a range of design-specific tools for qualitative papers too. A number of qualitative researchers have argued for a distinct set of criteria to natural scientific quantitative approaches by which to critique qualitative research (for example, Collins and Stockton, 2018; Dixon-Woods et al., 2004; Miyata and Kai, 2009). However, attempts to produce consensus on criteria for qualitative research appraisal have proved difficult. The UK's National Centre for Social Research (Spencer et al., 2003) produced a framework for assessing qualitative research, by drawing on 29 existing frameworks and conducting interviews and a workshop with those active in the field. The resulting tool they produced is useful but is lengthy and potentially unwieldy, consisting of 18 questions, over 7 pages. However, some means of determining the quality of qualitative studies is needed and so we should perhaps regard such criteria as guides to good practice rather than rigid requirements for every paper.

QUALITATIVE CRITIQUING TOOLS

As with quantitative research we have both generic and specific critical appraisal tools for each of the different study designs. We have already looked at the CRAAP test in Chapter 5 and this can be applied equally to both quantitative and qualitative research papers.

Additionally, Greenhalgh (1997) suggested that there should be eight questions that we ask of any qualitative paper, and this provides a useful informal framework for critiquing qualitative research. The eight questions are as follows:

1. Did the paper describe an important clinical problem addressed by a clearly formulated question?
2. Was a qualitative approach appropriate?
3. How were the setting and the subjects selected?
4. What was the researcher's perspective and has this been taken into account?
5. What methods did the researcher use for collecting data – and are these described in enough detail?
6. What methods did the research use to analyse the data – and what quality control measures were implemented?
7. Are the results credible and if so, are they clinically important?
8. What conclusions were drawn and are they justified by the results?

Similarly, Dixon-Woods et al. (2004) evaluated existing frameworks for appraisal of qualitative papers and held extensive discussions within a multidisciplinary project team to develop a set of prompts for appraising qualitative papers as follows:

1. Are the research questions clear?
2. Are the research questions suited to qualitative enquiry?
3. Are the sampling, data collection and analysis clearly described?
4. Are the claims made supported by sufficient evidence?
5. Are the data, interpretation and conclusions clearly integrated?
6. And does the paper make a useful contribution?

In developing these they explicitly avoided commitments to particular methodological approaches, instead they tried to distinguish between aspects of reporting and aspects of study design and execution. They proposed these as prompts, rather than 'criteria', in order to raise awareness to a specific set of issues. Such prompts could be used alongside critiquing tools specific to different methods of data collection and qualitative methodologies.

FORMAL CRITIQUING TOOLS

As discussed in relation to quantitative research, a number of tools are available to help with critical appraisal. We will now look at a few examples of these. An additional example is included at Appendix 5.

Let us start this section by looking at the Centre for Evidence-Based Medicine at Oxford's Critical Appraisal of Qualitative Studies tool (see www.cebm. ox.ac.uk/resources/ebm-tools/critical-appraisal-tools). Scroll down the critical appraisal worksheets and open the critical appraisal of qualitative studies sheet. Not only does this list the areas that you should look at in a research paper but gives an indication as to where to find this information in the paper. Now find a qualitative paper relating to a topic of interest to you and make a critique of the paper using the Critical Appraisal of Qualitative Studies tool. How useful did you find the tool in making a judgement of the paper?

Activity 7.2

Now take the time to explore the same paper using the different qualitative critiquing tools listed below. You will see we start with the CASP tool, which we were introduced to in Chapter 5. Following each tool ask the same question as in Activity 7.2. How useful did you find the tool in making a judgement of the paper? Again, as identified previously, have good research books to hand so information can be checked or clarified along the way.

Activity 7.3

- *Critical Appraisal Tools for the Evaluation of Published Studies.* Called the CASP (Critical Appraisal Skills Programme) Tools of the Public Health Research Unit of the National Health Service (UK), it contains separate study evaluation tools for systematic reviews, randomised control trials, economic evaluation studies, qualitative studies, cohort studies, case control studies and diagnostic test studies (see https://casp-uk.net/casp-tools-checklists/). Again, you are looking for the CASP Qualitative Studies Checklist.
- *COREQ (Consolidated Criteria for Reporting Qualitative Research)* (see https://academic.oup.com/view-large/27217733). The COREQ checklist was published in 2007, synthesised 22 original sources, and is a 32-item checklist.
- *Evaluation Tool for Qualitative Studies* (Long et al., 2002). https://usir.salford.ac.uk/id/eprint/12970/1/Evaluation_Tool_for_Qualitative_Studies.pdf
- Checklist for Qualitative Research (JBI.Global, 2020). https://jbi.global/sites/default/files/2020-08/Checklist_for_Qualitative_Research.pdf

The best way to get an idea of the different tools that are available for qualitative papers, and what they comprise, is to try them, and ideally try a few on the same paper. It really is a case of finding one that suits you. The author found over a hundred different tools when researching this chapter.

KEY AREAS TO CONSIDER WHEN CRITIQUING QUALITATIVE RESEARCH

The important thing to remember is that critiquing tools are just tools. They are aids, or prompts, to help you work systematically through a process so that you treat each paper the same. Just as important is to know what you are looking for and why. The following sections look at the main areas for consideration common to the tools above when critiquing a qualitative research paper.

A warning about the usage of terms. The differences between the various qualitative research designs can be difficult to understand at first. This is not helped by diversity in the use of terms among qualitative writers. The differences are quite subtle and are often concerned with the philosophical or other stance of the researchers and funders, the original research question, the people or situations being studied and the way the data are analysed, interpreted and presented. The important thing when getting to grips with qualitative research methodology is to read around the topic.

Research question and aims

Qualitative research normally will have a research question and not a hypothesis, as the intention is to generate understanding in relation to a phenomenon, not to predict a relationship between variables. The research question can take two forms (Cormack et al., 2015):

1. Interrogative – namely, a statement phrased as a question, e.g. 'What is the lived experience of people admitted to hospital following a suicide attempt?'
2. Declarative – namely, a statement which 'declares' the purpose of the study, e.g. 'It is intended to study the experience of people admitted to hospital following a suicide attempt.'

The best research questions are short and clearly identify a specific area of study. The question should set the scene for the research design that will allow the question to be answered. Some researchers will pose a series of questions while others identify a series of aims in relation to the question asked. The research question and aims should have the same intentions.

Literature review

An extensive literature review is not always the starting point of qualitative research. Often, only sufficient literature to provide a focus for the study will be considered. In phenomenological research the literature may not be reviewed until after the data have been collected and analysed. In grounded theory the literature is reviewed at various points throughout the data collection process and is used as a comparison for the interim research findings. This lack of initial literature review is to ensure that the analysis of the data is not influenced by what is already known about the topic. However, there is an expectation that the findings will be considered in light of the available literature, so that the study can be compared with other work and any issues regarding the **transferability** of findings to other settings can be identified.

Methodology

The chosen methodology should enable the research question to be answered. If the question asks about the meaning of something or an individual's experience, then you would expect to see a phenomenological design. If the stated aim is to investigate issues related to culture – beliefs, values, social norms – then an ethnographic approach would be more appropriate. There should be a match between what the researcher wants to know and the methodology used to answer the question. Table 7.2 gives an idea of the methodologies expected to be seen in relation to particular areas of study.

Reflexivity

While researcher involvement in the research process is a central tenet of qualitative research, there is also an expectation that researchers will discuss their beliefs, values, ideas and personal biases relating to the topic they are exploring, and this is usually given in the form of a reflective account. This reflexivity is seen as having two purposes. First, it makes the investigators aware of how their own beliefs may influence the data collection and interpretation. Having explored their own perspectives it is normally expected that researchers will put aside their beliefs in what is termed as **bracketing**. Here, researchers are expected not to make judgements about the appropriateness of what they see or hear, instead being open to what the data reveal rather than imposing their own beliefs on it. The second aspect relates to acknowledging that the researcher is part of the research process and ensures that the reader is aware of this.

> Identify an area you would be interested in researching. Write a short reflective piece identifying what beliefs and values you have in relation to the area and how that might impact on any research you undertook.
>
> **Activity 7.4**

However, while this process is an integral part of qualitative research, often the reflective account is missing from published work. The word limits imposed by journal publishers on authors of papers frequently result in this aspect being left out. When this is the case, the only insight given into the researchers' perspectives and backgrounds in terms of the research phenomenon is gained through examining their qualifications and job titles given at the beginning of the article.

Ethical issues

As identified in Chapter 5, all health service research requires ethical approval; however, the nature of qualitative research brings a distinct set of ethical issues into view. The interpersonal nature of most qualitative research (i.e. that the researcher and participants are in direct contact and form a close, albeit brief, trusting relationship) requires the researcher to be aware of any possible emotional impact the research may have on participants.

Streubert and Carpenter (2010) identify various aspects that are important in qualitative research, and these are areas you should consider when doing a critical appraisal:

1. Informed consent – within qualitative research participants must be allowed to withdraw this consent at any point. 'Process informed' consent is often adopted, where a participant's consent will be re-evaluated at various points within the study and involvement stopped if required.
2. Confidentiality and anonymity – the one-to-one interaction between participant and researcher means that anonymity is not possible in the same way as in quantitative research; the researcher will obviously know where the data came from. However, confidentiality can and must be maintained, with every effort made to ensure that participants are not recognisable in the data used to support descriptions of results.
3. The researcher–participant relationship – the researcher must be clear about the boundaries of this relationship. This is a particular issue for healthcare professionals, who may find their role as care provider conflicting with their role of researcher.
4. Sensitive issues – some of the issues discussed during data collection can be distressing for the participants and/or the researcher. It is important that the researcher identifies mechanisms for dealing with such issues and how participants will be supported following data collection.

Activity 7.5

Imagine you are conducting a research study discussing a topic which may cause the participants to become distressed. What support do you think it would be important to offer to the participants?

Sampling/participant selection

In qualitative research, sampling can occur at several stages, both while collecting data and while interpreting and reporting on it. Sampling while collecting data for qualitative research is not the same as sampling in quantitative research because researchers are not interested in being able to generalise at a statistical level – instead the key is purposive or strategic sampling.

Individuals are usually selected to participate in particular research because they will have had experience of or are involved in the phenomenon being studied. For instance, if the research question is 'What is the lived experience of people with schizophrenia?' the people selected to participate in the study would be people with schizophrenia, as only they would be able to describe their experiences.

As the intention with qualitative research is to gain a greater understanding of the area of interest, not to generalise findings, randomised sampling is not an issue here. There are various approaches to sampling the population of interest:

- Convenience – the most conveniently available people are selected, those who are closest to hand and relevant to the phenomenon of interest.
- Snowballing – a form of convenience sampling where having identified an informant to tell you about the phenomenon, they then identify someone else.
- Purposive or purposeful – selecting people who can tell you about the research phenomenon; this approach tends to be used in phenomenological studies.
- Theoretical – a framework is created in which the principal concepts related to the study are identified and individuals are selected to participate who are judged to have theoretical purpose/relevance; the researcher clearly states the basic types of participants to be included and how these individuals will facilitate the collection of appropriate data to describe the phenomenon. This approach is most often seen in grounded theory.

Sample sizes in qualitative research are normally small in comparison to quantitative research. It is not unusual to see research conducted on just 10 people. The nature of the data collected and subsequent analysis makes large samples almost impossible to handle. For example, one 45-minute interview can produce 30 pages of transcribed information. Just 10 participants would therefore result in around 300 pages requiring analysis. The aim of qualitative research is to reduce this huge amount of information to a manageable size without losing the participants' intended meaning.

The sample size is largely decided by the type of research, the quality of the information provided by the participants and the sampling approach used. Often, qualitative researchers talk about reaching **data saturation**, particularly in grounded theory. This is the point where no new information is being collected from participants and is usually the point where data collection stops. So, for example, if data saturation is reached after interviewing 12 people then no further interviews will be conducted.

Data collection

We are asking the same questions of qualitative papers as we asked of quantitative papers. For example, was the method appropriate for the research question, for the approach, or for the type of data? Who conducted the study and why? What data were collected? Where were the data collected? When were they collected? How often were they collected? How were they collected? How many were collected? (and not collected), and who collected the data? How were the data analysed? Who analysed them and how might that impact on the interpretation? What sense did they make of the findings? What were the recommendations that came from the research? How useful is this to my practice?

There are various forms of data collection available to the qualitative researcher, but most involve the collection of 'words' in some shape or form. Table 7.3 provides an overview of the main types of activity. In appraising a study it is important to consider whether the form of data collection used will provide the researcher with the most appropriate data.

It is essential that a study identifies how the information from participants was recorded. Many researchers will use audio recording devices, some may incorporate video recording to ensure that non-verbal responses are captured. While field notes are useful and add to the picture, they tend to be incomplete and do not enable the researcher to revisit the interaction in its original form.

Table 7.3   Types of data collection

Type	Description
Interviews	Unstructured – no prepared questions apart from asking them to talk about the phenomenon of interest
	Semi-structured – a guide asking open questions related to the areas of interest, prepared in advance
	(Structured – not used in qualitative research)
Focus groups	Group interviews, 6–12 people discussing a topic
Observation	Participant observation – the researcher is part of the group and is involved in its activities
	Observer-participant – the researcher generally observes and may interview members of the group and may also participate in some activities
	Complete observer – no interaction between observer and participant
Field notes	In ethnography these involve documenting observations and narratives
	In phenomenology these may involve recording individual expressions and other aspects not captured by audio recording of interviews
Diaries	Unstructured – where people are asked simply to record their thoughts and feelings
	Structured – where people are asked to write about specific aspects
Documentation	Patient notes, historical records, health service documentation and records; published and unpublished works

Data analysis

Polit and Beck (2018) propose that qualitative data analysis is more difficult to do than quantitative analysis but easier to understand, which is a bonus for those who are critiquing rather than doing the research. However, it is not always easy to fully appraise the findings, as you cannot know if the authors have given an appropriate representation of participants' narratives.

Qualitative analysis usually involves some sort of content analysis where researchers create categories and themes from the data. As these categories are created, a coding system is then developed which allows statements made by participants to be grouped together in particular categories. Once such categories have been identified these may then be further grouped into themes. Data can be handled manually or analysed using computer-assisted qualitative data analysis systems (CAQDAS) such as NVivo. However, as there are a number of approaches to qualitative research, the content analysis takes various forms. Note this lack of a universal approach can make it difficult to critically appraise the work.

When critically appraising a qualitative analysis you are looking to see if the author has given you enough information to make a judgement as to whether the analysis has been conducted in an appropriate way. There are a number of basic tenets you would expect to be described:

1. Data transcription – how the data are translated from audio to a written form; what steps were taken to ensure data were of the best quality, including identification of problems related to transcription (e.g. background noise, poor tape quality, participant's voice inaudible).
2. Identification of tool used for analysis – a number of tools would be available and the one chosen should be appropriate to the research methodology. For example, you would not expect a grounded theory methodology to include Colaizzi's (1978) approach, which is specific to phenomenology. The researcher involved should clearly identify the approach taken and you should be able to follow this step-by-step through the paper.
3. Interpretation – this occurs at the same time as the analysis, as the researcher reads and re-reads the data and the codes, categories/themes and tries to make sense of the data. The writer should give details of how the interpretation was arrived at.

Throughout the course of qualitative analysis, the analyst should be asking and re-asking the following questions:

*   What patterns and common themes emerge in responses dealing with specific items? How do these patterns (or lack thereof) help to illuminate the broader study question(s)?
*   Are there any deviations from these patterns? If yes, are there any factors that might explain these atypical responses?
*   What interesting stories emerge from the responses? How can these stories help to illuminate the broader study question(s)?
*   Do any of these patterns or findings suggest that additional data may need to be collected? Do any of the study questions need to be revised?
*   Do the patterns that emerge corroborate the findings of any corresponding qualitative analyses that have been conducted? If not, what might explain these discrepancies?

Issues of rigour

Streubert and Carpenter (2010) suggested that decisions as to the rigour of a particular research study are a 'judgement call'. They go on to suggest that two fundamental characteristics of qualitative research should be present when making this judgement as to whether it meets the implicit goal of providing an accurate account of participants' perspective:

1. Is there adequate attention to the collection of information?
2. Is there confirmation of the accuracy of the information?

In focusing on the above areas (see Table 7.4) in the research as part of the critique we are being asked to make a judgement as to the quality and values of the research. Stenfors et al. (2020) offer a useful framework to appraise the trustworthiness and therefore quality of qualitative study (see Table 7.5)

Remember, in critically appraising qualitative papers we are seeking to do the same thing as we do with quantitative papers. We are seeking to assess the usefulness or the evidence. We are trying to work out whether we can trust the findings and conclusions of a study, and also whether or not it is relevant to our clinical practice.

Table 7.4   Criteria for assessing rigour of qualitative research

Criteria	Ways of identifying if criteria are met
Credibility	Findings returned to participants for confirmation that they are a true representation of their experiences
	All data are accounted for, including instances where the data are inconsistent with other findings
	Triangulation
Dependability	Reporting of unexpected events and how dealt with
	Recording methods ensured quality of data
	Triangulation
Confirmability	Evidence of reflexivity
	Provision of an 'audit trail' to enable the thought and decision-making processes to be identified (a research diary or recording mechanisms within CAQDAS)
Transferability	Providing a full description of the research setting and participants
	Identifying that the findings have relevance to similar situations
	Theoretical triangulation
Authenticity	The reality of the participants' lives is conveyed, enabling you to understand the range of feelings experienced by those involved

Table 7.5   Accessing trustworthiness

Criteria	What it means	How to recognise it
Credibility	The research findings are plausible and trustworthy	There is alignment between theory, research question, data collection, analysis and results. Sampling strategy, the depth and volume of data, and the analytical steps taken, are appropriate within that framework.
Dependability	The extent to which the research could be replicated in similar conditions	There is sufficient information provided such that another researcher could follow the same procedural steps, albeit possibly reaching different conclusions.
Confirmability	There is a clear link or relationship between the data and the findings	The researchers show how they made their findings through detailed descriptions and the use of quotes.
Transferability	Findings may be transferred to another setting, context or group	Detailed description of the context in which the research was performed and how this shaped the findings.
Reflexivity	A continual process of engaging with and articulating the place of the researcher and the context of the research	Explanations of how reflexivity was embedded and supported in the research process.

(Adapted from Stenfors et al., 2020)

Summary

- There are a number of approaches to qualitative research, each with their own theoretical and philosophical underpinning, generally focusing on how people describe their experiences, perspectives, understanding and beliefs/values.
- Ethical issues take a particular form in qualitative research.
- Sample sizes in qualitative research are normally small in comparison to quantitative research. Individuals are usually invited to participate in particular research because they have experience or are involved in the phenomenon being studied.
- There are various forms of data collection available to the qualitative researcher, but most of them involve the collecting of 'words' in some shape or form and analysis involves some sort of content analysis where the researcher creates categories and themes from the data.

FURTHER READING

Ryan, F., Coughlan, M. and Cronin, P. (2007) 'Step-by-step guide to critiquing research. Part 2: qualitative research', *British Journal of Nursing, 16*(12): 738–45.

USEFUL WEBLINKS

Critical Appraisal Skills Programme: provides a range of resources to help with developing the skills associated with EBP. Also provides a range of critical appraisal tools. www.casp-uk.net

QualPage: provides resources and information related to qualitative research. The methods section provides an overview of different qualitative methodologies. www.qualitativeresearch.uga.edu/QualPage

8

Systematic Reviews and Evidence-based Practice

Marishona Ortega

Learning Outcomes

By the end of the chapter, you will be able to:

- discuss the systematic review process and its key features;
- identify key areas for consideration when critically appraising systematic reviews;
- identify issues to be considered when assessing the rigour of systematic reviews.

INTRODUCTION

> The notion of systematic review – looking at the totality of evidence – is quietly one of the most important innovations in medicine over the past 30 years. (Goldacre, 2011: xi)

The explosion of literature related to healthcare has made it almost impossible for any practitioner to keep abreast of all current research findings. As has already been mentioned in Chapter 4, the US National Library of Medicine added nearly 1 million records to MEDLINE in 2020 alone (US National Library of Medicine, 2020). It was even estimated that by 2020, it would only take 73 days for medical knowledge to double (Densen, 2011). We are perhaps reaching a point where relevant knowledge is increasing at a rate greater than we can absorb (Chamberlain, 2020) and therefore the ability for nurses and health professionals to look at 'the totality of evidence' through **systematic reviews** (Goldacre, 2011) is increasingly important.

As identified in Chapter 1, in many ways EBP is seen as having its origins in Professor Archie Cochrane's criticisms of the medical profession for its failure to use the body of evidence available to it in an appropriate way and his call for the development of up-to-date 'critical summaries' of all randomised controlled trials (RCTs) relevant to a specialty or sub-specialty (Cochrane, 1979). This ultimately led to the formation of the Cochrane Collaboration in 1993 and creation of the Cochrane Database of Systematic Reviews in 1995. Prior to the emergence of EBP, summaries of studies more frequently appeared in the form of what Greenhalgh (2019) terms as 'journalistic reviews'. Here papers were reviewed, selected and analysed in an ad hoc manner, subject to the vagaries of the person conducting the literature review. In many ways this left any interpretation provided open to accusations of bias, and the lack of a systematic approach gave the reader little evidence on which to consider the credibility of the findings. However, since the advent of EBP, systematic reviews have become more prevalent; in the decade since its launch in 2011, 100,000 systematic reviews have been registered on PROSPERO, the international database of prospectively registered systematic reviews in health and social care, welfare, public health, education, crime, justice, and international development, where there is a health-related outcome (Centre for Reviews and Dissemination, 2021). Although systematic reviews employ rigorous methods, which are explicit and reproducible, critical appraisal of systematic reviews is just as important as appraising single studies before implementing any results into your practice.

This chapter will consider the methods and approaches used in systematic reviews and the areas to be considered when critically appraising this form of evidence.

WHAT IS A SYSTEMATIC REVIEW?

Systematic reviews provide a rigorous review of research findings in relation to a specific question, saving nurses and other healthcare professionals the time and effort it would take to search and appraise a large body of evidence in order to keep up-to-date with knowledge in their field. Parahoo defines systematic reviews as 'the rigorous and systematic search, selection, appraisal, synthesis and summary of the findings of primary research studies in order to answer a specific question' (2014: 123). One of the key differences between a systematic review and a traditional literature review is that they start with a well-defined question and the methods used are transparent and reproducible with steps taken to minimise bias; they also help to connect health professionals to high-quality evidence. Systematic reviews are often used as a starting point for the development of clinical practice guidelines (Moher et al., 2009; National Institute for Health and Care Excellence [NICE], 2020). While it is not expected that health professionals in general undertake systematic reviews (they can be both complex and time consuming to complete), there is a need to be able to recognise, appraise and evaluate their usefulness for practice.

Systematic reviews are fundamental to EBP, as can be seen in the Evidence-Based Health Care (EBHC) Pyramid 5.0 (Alper and Haynes, 2016), where they form one of the levels of sound evidence on which nurses and other healthcare professionals can base practice. Greenhalgh (2019) lists a number of advantages that systematic reviews have over single studies, including the fact that they allow practitioners to assimilate large amounts of information quickly, which speeds up the decision-making process.

Systematic review is a term that is often used interchangeably with **meta–analysis**, but as you will see from the discussion below the two are not the same. Systematic reviews have previously been primarily associated with quantitative research, but systematic reviews of qualitative research with an accompanying **synthesis** of the qualitative findings are becoming increasingly common. The value of qualitative systematic reviews is that health professionals can move beyond questions of 'does it work?' to questions about 'how do people feel about this?' (Garside, 2014). Methods for qualitative systematic reviews are still developing, with the Cochrane Library only publishing their first qualitative review in 2013 (Glenton et al., 2013) in what was described as a milestone for the organisation (Gülmezoglu et al., 2013). There are also systematic reviews that use a mixed methods approach which integrate both qualitative and quantitative review questions, research designs and techniques for collecting and analysing data, although this approach is still an 'emerging field of enquiry' (Lizarondo et al., 2020). One advantage of mixed methods reviews is that by maximising their findings they have a greater ability to inform both policy and practice in that they address not only questions of effectiveness (quantitative) but also of experience (qualitative) (Lizarondo et al., 2020; Pearson et al., 2015).

Following concerns raised about the clarity of reporting in systematic reviews (Moher et al., 2009), guidelines in the form of the PRISMA (Preferred Reporting Items for Systematic Reviews and Meta-Analyses) statement were developed as 'an evidence-based minimum set of items for reporting in systematic reviews and meta-analyses' (PRISMA, 2021a). The original PRISMA statement of 2009 has recently been updated and provides new guidance that reflects advances in review methodology and terminology (Page et al., 2021). It is endorsed by Cochrane and the Centre for Reviews and Dissemination (PRISMA, 2021b) as well as nearly 200 journals and systematic review organisations (Page et al., 2021). Since launching, a number of extensions to the statement have been developed to take into account different aspects or types of review; the latest being PRISMA-S, which provides guidance on the reporting of literature searches in systematic reviews (Rethlefsen et al., 2021).

A number of tools have also been developed to ensure the quality of qualitative syntheses such as the ENTREQ (Enhancing Transparency in Reporting the Synthesis of Qualitative Research) statement. This was devised to report the stages most commonly associated with the synthesis of qualitative health research: searching and selecting qualitative research, quality appraisal, and methods for synthesising qualitative findings (Tong et al., 2012).

Activity 8.1

Visit the PRISMA website (www.prisma-statement.org). Identify two of the items on the 27-item PRISMA 2020 checklist provided in relation to a systematic review or meta-analysis that you would like to learn more about. Create an action plan on how you will develop your learning in relation to these two areas.

Systematic reviews are a form of research, often termed **secondary research** in that they are based on research already undertaken; however, their strength lies in their ability to reduce potential bias, and improve the reliability and accuracy of conclusions

(Akobeng, 2005). Cochrane produce systematic reviews, which are widely recognised as the gold standard, where they 'seek to collate evidence that fits pre-specified eligibility criteria in order to answer a specific research question' (Chandler et al., 2021). The process of 'collating' this evidence is a systematic process – Box 8.1 identifies the steps associated with systematic reviews.

TYPES OF SYSTEMATIC REVIEWS

Systematic reviews and the subject of evidence synthesis is an evolving one with new methods being developed and new terminology coming into use. Sutton et al. (2019) describe a 'review family' and identified 48 separate review types, which were categorised into seven families. These families include traditional, systematic, qualitative, mixed method and purpose-specific reviews but also rapid reviews as well as reviews of reviews. Rapid reviews follow a simplified systematic review process to produce information in a timely manner (Tricco et al., 2015); a review of reviews also follows the same methods as a systematic review but will only include reviews and other evidence syntheses (Sutton et al., 2019).

Another relatively recent development is that of the Living Systematic Review (LSR) defined by Cochrane as a 'systematic review which is continually updated, incorporating relevant new evidence as it becomes available' (Cochrane Community, 2019). LSRs have been particularly relevant during the COVID-19 pandemic in a rapidly evolving context where new clinical trials were being registered every week due to the urgency of the situation (Maguire and Guérin, 2020). The *BMJ* published their first LSR in April 2020 evaluating prognostic models in COVID-19 (Wynants et al., 2020) and the concept is seen as gathering momentum (Macdonald et al., 2020). Due to the ongoing nature of reviewing and synthesising evidence, LSRs can facilitate 'living recommendations' and assist with the decision-making process (Mavergames and Elliott, n.d.).

As previously mentioned, Sutton et al. (2019) distinguish systematic reviews of quantitative evidence and qualitative evidence as two distinct families. The basic steps for both types of review are generally the same; however, differences occur when synthesising the evidence, which will be explored later in this chapter. The key features of systematic reviews, whether quantitative or qualitative, are that they are explicit in their methods and statement of objectives and that the methodology employed is 'transparent and reproducible' (Greenhalgh, 2019: 117).

Box 8.1   Systematic review process

1. Formulate and frame question.
2. Search for and select relevant studies.
3. Extract data.
4. Assess the quality of the studies.
5. Synthesise and present results.
6. Conclude and make recommendations.

FORMULATE AND FRAME QUESTION

The development of a review protocol should be the first step when undertaking a systematic review. The protocol gives direction and it should describe the rationale, hypothesis and methodology of the planned review. There are various checklists available to facilitate the reporting of protocols, with one example being PRISMA-P (Moher et al., 2015). Registering the protocol in an international resource such as PROSPERO at www.crd. york.ac.uk/prospero can help to reduce duplication in that it provides a comprehensive listing of reviews and their status. It can also reduce possible reporting bias by allowing comparison of the completed review with what was planned in the protocol. The protocols for all Cochrane reviews are also made available via the Cochrane Database of Systematic Reviews at www.cochranelibrary.com.

All systematic reviews should have a clearly identifiable and well-formulated question; this is sometimes presented in the PICO format or a variation of this (see Chapter 4 for some examples) depending on the type of review being undertaken. Without this, the reviewer and the reader will not be able to decide whether relevant papers are included. While a particular question such as 'Does eating breakfast improve cognitive functioning in children?' may initially sound appropriate; when you start to pull it apart and consider each aspect, such as what is meant by children (all under-18s or a specific group?), breakfast (a slice of toast or a 'full English'?) and cognitive functioning (alertness, memory, understanding, completion of tests?), then it becomes apparent that the need for clear identification of the various aspects is key to the whole process.

As with any research, the objectives should be clearly stated and flow from the question. The inclusion/exclusion criteria identify the limits of the review and give a clear indication of what is to be included in the review and what is not. Sound justifications are expected to be present for the setting of the limits as well as a clear exploration of the implications of these for the review.

Search for and select relevant studies

The methods used to identify the studies relevant to a particular systematic review are a fundamental issue when assessing its rigour. The search for literature is a 'crucial component' of a systematic review in that the data that are analysed and the subsequent results are entirely dependent on the quality of the search, which should be robust, reproducible and which minimises bias (Rethlefsen et al., 2021). When undertaking a systematic review, the reviewers must ensure that all studies relevant to the topic are identified. This will require the creation of a comprehensive search strategy, which is highly sensitive, thus ensuring that any studies relevant to the review are retrieved. As the validity of the review is reliant on the quality of the search strategy, it is essential that it is clearly reported in the final review. The same principles discussed in Chapter 4 apply when identifying what search terms and databases are appropriate. However, it is worth noting that for qualitative systematic reviews, the search process can present challenges due to poor indexing, non-informative titles and abstracts as well as the fact that qualitative evidence is also more likely to be found in book chapters, theses and grey literature (Noyes et al., 2021).

According to Booth et al. (2016a) the search methods that should be employed in a systematic review are:

- database searching;
- hand searching of journals;
- bibliographic searching such as checking reference lists for potential sources or citation searching;
- searching for grey literature;
- identifying ongoing research;
- contacting experts.

When critically appraising a systematic review, it is important to consider whether all relevant sources of literature have been searched as this may have an impact on the rigour of the review.

List databases and other sources of information you would consider key to finding literature related to your own area of practice.

Activity 8.2

Extract data

The method of summarising the evidence or data extraction should be clearly identified. The purpose of data extraction is to extract the findings from each study in a consistent manner in order to facilitate synthesis. The methods will vary depending on the purpose of the review, but it is important that it is undertaken in as reliable and unbiased a way as possible. There are different types of software available to assist with these processes (see Table 8.1). For quantitative reviews, information about the studies is usually presented in the form of tables identifying:

- study characteristics, e.g. aims, objectives, inclusion and exclusion criteria;
- participant characteristics, e.g. age, gender, ethnicity;
- intervention – details of the exact form of intervention (and control) and how it was delivered (e.g. routes, dosages, timing, instructions for delivery);
- outcome measures – the reviewers should clearly identify what outcome measures are under consideration;
- results of study analysis.

In relation to qualitative reviews it is expected that a study's methodology (phenomenology, ethnography, etc.), cultural features (age, socioeconomic group and ethnicity) and form of data collection (interview, focus group, etc.) will be clearly recorded.

Table 8.1   A selection of systematic review software/tools

Systematic Review Toolbox	A web-based catalogue of tools that support various tasks within the systematic review and wider evidence synthesis process **http://systematicreviewtools.com**
Review Manager RevMan 5 (desktop) RevMan Web (online)	Software used for preparing and maintaining Cochrane reviews **https://training.cochrane.org/online-learning/core-software-cochrane-reviews/revman**
GRADEPro GDT	Software developed to support the creation of summary of findings tables for systematic reviews, health technology assessments and guidelines **https://gradepro.org**
EPPI-reviewer	Software developed to support all types of literature review, including systematic reviews, meta-analyses, 'narrative' reviews and meta-ethnographies **https://eppi.ioe.ac.uk**
JBI SUMARI	Produced by JBI (formerly known as the Joanna Briggs Institute) this software is designed to facilitate the entire review process, including protocol development study selection, critical appraisal, data extraction and synthesis **https://sumari.jbi.global**
Covidence	Software for importing citations, screening titles and abstracts, undertaking risk of bias assessment and data extraction **www.covidence.org**
Rayyan	Free software for screening titles and abstracts and includes features such as text mining tools **www.rayyan.ai**

These tables will allow you to compare various studies and help you to make a judgement as to the rigour of the systematic review. If a table indicates there is significant heterogeneity within quantitative studies, then it is unlikely that the results will be subjected to meta-analysis. It is possible to synthesise heterogeneous qualitative studies and this is discussed later in the chapter. Where it is not possible or appropriate to pool data in the form of a meta-analysis, a narrative integration or written summary of findings should be provided.

Assessing the quality of the studies

The quality of the literature to be included in a systematic review should be assessed and some form of appraisal of each study should be undertaken. (See Chapters 6 and 7 of this book for further details on critiquing the evidence.) Consideration should be given to the methodological quality of a study, including an assessment of the possibility of bias in its design and analysis (Aromataris et al., 2015). Study design is often used as a 'general marker of study quality' (Khan et al., 2011: 39); for example, Cochrane systematic reviews which assess the effectiveness of a healthcare intervention will generally only include RCTs. Therefore, only studies meeting a minimum standard will be considered for inclusion. Assessing quality in qualitative research is a contested area with qualitative researchers failing to agree as to what constitutes 'validity' or 'quality' (Garside, 2014). However, in the *Cochrane Handbook for Systematic Reviews of Interventions* (Noyes et al., 2021), the advice is that assessing methodological strengths and limitations is essential and it recommends the use of validated tools such as the CASP checklist for qualitative research (Critical Appraisal Skills Programme, 2018).

Consideration must also be given as to what measures have been taken to minimise bias, which could affect data interpretation and possibly lead to distorted inferences being drawn (Acosta et al., 2020). A bias as defined in the *Cochrane Handbook* is 'a systematic error, or deviation from the truth, in results' (Boutron et al., 2021: section 7.1). A number of tools, including scales and checklists, are available to help identify the risk of bias in both randomised and non-randomised studies; one example is Cochrane's revised Risk of Bias Tool for randomised trials (RoB 2) (Sterne et al., 2019). RoB 2 can be used to assess, through signalling questions, bias in five domains, including different aspects of trial design, conduct and reporting. Whichever method is employed should be identified and appropriate to the type of research under consideration.

The use of at least two reviewers is also the norm in systematic reviews, which can help to minimise bias and hopefully reduce the chance that eligible studies are excluded. They should independently review each study identified and reach agreement as to their eligibility for inclusion in the review. All steps in this process should be transparent and recorded. The selection process can be very time-consuming, so the use of software (see Table 8.1 for examples) can assist with this.

Synthesise and present results

Synthesis is the 'collation, combination and summary of the findings of individual studies included in the systematic review' (Centre for Reviews and Dissemination, 2009). Different methods will be employed depending on whether quantitative or qualitative evidence is being combined.

Systematic reviews have traditionally assessed the effectiveness of healthcare interventions by summarising and synthesising relevant quantitative studies such as RCTs and where appropriate include a meta-analysis, which involves the 'pooling' or aggregation of results from 'like' studies to create a larger data set for analysis (Pearson et al., 2007: 92). A meta-analysis can also be seen as giving an overall picture of the effectiveness of an intervention. There is broad consensus as to these methods, which will be detailed below; however, the same cannot be said for qualitative evidence. The synthesis of qualitative evidence is more complex; it is a rapidly evolving area of study with different schools of thought leading to different approaches, namely aggregative and interpretive (Gough et al., 2017). Polit and Beck (2020) consider that most qualitative systematic reviews will have elements of both aggregation and interpretation and the method of synthesis employed will ultimately be dependent on the type of question being addressed as well as the reviewers' philosophical leanings. Booth et al. (2016b) identified over 20 different methods for qualitative evidence synthesis; although some methods have developed further and have been subject to more testing than others. The umbrella term to describe all these different methods (and the term preferred by the Cochrane Qualitative Methods & Implementation Group) is Qualitative Evidence Synthesis (QES). Two of these approaches, specifically **meta-synthesis** and meta-aggregation, will be explored below.

Meta-analysis

Meta-analysis is defined by Greenhalgh (2019: 125) as 'a statistical synthesis of the numerical results of several trials that all addressed the same question'. It enables the bringing together of results for studies that are said to be homogeneous in nature – considering the same outcome of the same intervention, on the same population – in an objective way. The effect of combining the results of a number of smaller studies by way of meta-analysis can improve precision and the ability to answer questions not asked by individual studies and settle controversies arising from apparently conflicting studies or to generate new hypotheses (Deeks et al., 2021).

Meta-analysis normally has two stages (Deeks et al., 2021):

1. A summary statistic is calculated for each study, to describe the observed intervention (treatment) effect in the same way for every study. See Table 8.2 for examples of common measures.
2. The summary or combined intervention (treatment) effect is calculated as a weighted average of intervention effects estimated in the individual studies.

Table 8.2   Treatment effect measures

Measure	Description
Odds ratio (OR)	OR is the ratio of the odds of an event or outcome in the intervention group to the odds of an outcome in the control group.
	An OR of 1 indicates no difference between comparison groups.
	For an undesirable outcome an OR < 1 indicates the intervention is effective in reducing the odds of that outcome.
Relative risk (RR)	Also known as risk ratio. RR is the ratio of the risk in the intervention group to the risk in the control group.
	A RR of 1 indicates no difference between comparison groups.
	For an undesirable outcome, an RR < 1 indicates the intervention is effective in reducing the risk of that outcome.
Risk difference (RD)	Also known as Absolute Risk Reduction (ARR). In comparative studies, it is the difference in event rates between two groups.
Number needed to treat (NNT)	NNT is the number of patients who need to be treated to prevent one undesirable outcome. In an individual study it is the inverse of RD.
Number needed to harm (NNH)	NNH is the number of patients who need to be treated for one additional patient to experience an episode of harm (adverse effect, complication, etc.)

Source: Khan et al., 2011. CRC Press. Reproduced with kind permission of Taylor & Francis.

The reviewers begin by deciding which of the outcome measures of the studies reviewed are to be used for the meta-analysis – in most studies a number of outcomes are measured, although only some of these may be of interest to the reviewers. The findings in relation to these outcomes are presented as treatment effect measures, which identify the strength and direction of the relationship between the independent and dependent variables.

The reviewers will also identify what is known as statistical heterogeneity – that is, how diverse the effects are across the various studies. This is usually demonstrated through the use of forest plot graphs – sometimes referred to as 'blobbograms' (see Figure 8.1 for an example).

A forest plot is a graphical representation of a meta-analysis. Each horizontal line represents the results of one study and the square or 'blob' in the middle of each line is the estimated treatment effect of the study (odds ratio, relative risk, etc.). The size of the blob represents the size of the effect, which is usually in proportion to the number of participants in the study; larger studies receive a greater weighting than smaller studies. The width of the line represents the 95% confidence interval of this treatment effect – as identified in Chapter 6, the wider the interval the less precise the estimate. The vertical line is the 'line of no effect' where the intervention group is no better or worse than the control group. In this example, if the confidence interval of a particular study crosses the 'line of no effect' it means that either there is no significant difference between treatment groups and/or the sample is too small to be confident that there is an effect. The heterogeneity of studies can be instantly assessed in forest plot graphs as the more scattered the lines, the more heterogeneous the results. The more heterogeneous the results, the less confidence there is in the ability to use the results in practice.

The diamond below all the horizontal lines represents the pooled effect of combining all the studies. The diamond's position reflects whether overall there is confidence that one treatment is better than the other. On the line means that for the average person there is little choice between the two, while to the left of the line identifies one is better than the other.

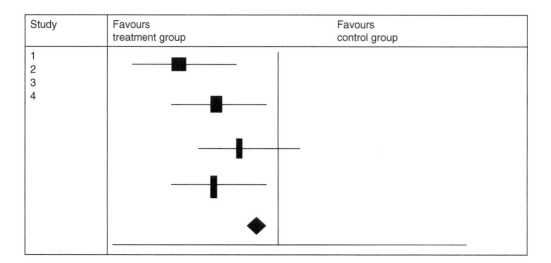

Figure 8.1   Forest plot graph

If the studies are seen as homogeneous and heterogeneity of treatment effects are identified between studies, Khan et al. (2011: 56) suggest that this may be due to differences in the characteristics of populations, interventions, outcomes or study design. For example, if in one study the sample of older people included those between the ages of 65 and 80 years and in another the sample was made up of those aged over 80, that would represent a heterogeneous population and may explain why differences in the effect of an intervention were seen. Where none of the above is apparent, Khan et al. (2011) suggest that heterogeneity may be a result of **publication bias**. This type of bias occurs due to a tendency in some areas for only positive results to be published, and when using such findings for systematic reviews a bias towards effectiveness is likely. It is expected that the reviewers should explore this possibility.

It may be the case that individual studies are too small to produce precise effects, but the precision is improved by combining them in a meta-analysis (Khan et al., 2011: 57). The Cochrane logo is a representation of an example of this pooling which identified significance. It represents a meta-analysis of seven RCTs related to the effect of corticosteroids on women expected to give birth prematurely. The first RCT on this subject was published in 1972; however, it wasn't until the publication of a systematic review in 1989 by Crowley that the effectiveness of this treatment was finally recognised (Crowley, 1989). This led to more widespread use of corticosteroids on women at risk of pre-term birth, thus probably saving thousands of premature babies (Cochrane Community, 2017).

Activity 8.3

Visit the Cochrane website at www.cochrane.org and view the logo.

A sensitivity analysis is usually undertaken to identify any changes in the original data that may have occurred as a result of pooling. This involves re-analysing data from different perspectives to see if this has an impact on the results. If substantial changes are reported to have occurred as a result of pooling data, then caution should be taken in applying the results to your own area of practice.

Activity 8.4

Visit the Cochrane Library at www.cochranelibrary.com and access a systematic review relevant to your own area of practice and familiarise yourself with the organisation and layout of a systematic review and meta-analysis.

Meta-synthesis

Meta-synthesis is derived from the Greek words *meta* meaning 'denoting change, transformation, permutation, or substitution' and *synthesis* meaning 'a body of things put together;

a complex whole made up of a number of parts or elements united' (*Oxford English Dictionary*, 2021). This suggests meta-synthesis is about putting together things in a way that goes beyond the features of the individual items and that it is a transformational process. Finlayson and Dixon (2008) have suggested it is the bringing together of the findings of qualitative research in an effort to provide a clearer picture of the phenomenon of interest. As Booth (2006: 422) states, with meta-synthesis 'the goal… is not aggregative in the sense of "adding studies together" as with a meta-analysis. On the contrary, it is interpretative in broadening understanding of a particular phenomenon.'

Lachal et al. (2017) suggest that the value of qualitative syntheses is now being recognised in that they allow the 'meanings, experiences and perspectives' of participants to be examined both deeply and broadly. Understanding people's experiences through qualitative evidence gives the patient/client or provider a voice in the healthcare decision-making process (Lockwood et al., 2020).

The processes involved with meta-synthesis are very similar to that of primary qualitative research and, as in any form of qualitative research, the reviewers are providing an interpretation of the findings. The process appears on the face of it to be a simple one, but in reality, is quite complex and requires a rigorous examination of the studies. The aim is to provide an accurate representation of the findings, which gives a full picture of the essential characteristics of the phenomenon under consideration. The specific approach used to achieve this is expected to be clearly outlined to enable you to judge the rigour of the process and the appropriateness of the review for application within an area of practice.

Whereas heterogeneity is an issue of great concern within meta-analysis it is less so within meta-synthesis (Evans and Pearson, 2001). In qualitative research heterogeneity is anticipated; the issue for reviewers is to ensure that differences are acknowledged, compared across studies and accounted for within the new interpretation.

Polit and Beck (2020) describe two approaches to meta-synthesis, which are outlined in Table 8.3.

Meta-aggregation

Aggregative reviews are similar to quantitative systematic reviews in that they involve the pooling of findings with the goal being to provide 'direct, usable guidance for action' (Polit and Beck, 2020: 298). JBI's guidance on qualitative evidence synthesis takes an aggregative approach, with the institute's preferred method being meta-aggregation. This highly structured method has the specific aim of delivering synthesised findings that will directly inform clinical decision making as well as policy development (Hannes and Lockwood, 2011).

The process of a qualitative systematic review following the meta-aggregation method will start with a clearly defined question; however, it is worth noting that instead of using the PICO framework (see Chapter 4 for further details), JBI recommend using PICo (**P**opulation, phenomenon of **I**nterest, **Co**ntext). The other processes that follow are very similar to those found in a quantitative systematic review. Synthesis in meta-aggregation is a three-step process, which starts with an extraction of findings from all included studies. The second step is to develop categories of findings (with at least two findings per category) and in the final step reviewers develop one or more synthesised findings of at

Table 8.3   Meta-synthesis approaches (Polit and Beck, 2020)

Approach	Description	Example
Noblit and Hare (1988) (Meta-ethnography)	• Consists of seven phases and focuses on constructing interpretations rather than descriptions. Considers how studies relate to each other (either reciprocal – directly comparable; refutational – in opposition to each other or alternatively in a line of argument) • Translating studies, ensuring main concepts are reflected • Synthesising the various translations into a comprehensible whole • Providing a narrative account of the synthesis	Dahl, B., Heinonen, K. and Bondas, T.E. (2020) 'From midwife-dominated to midwifery-led antenatal care: a meta-ethnography', *International Journal of Environmental Research and Public Health*, 17(23): 8946.
Sandelowski and Barroso (2007)	• Consists of two processes of synthesising qualitative research • Meta-summary is the 'quantitatively oriented aggregation of qualitative research findings that are themselves topical or thematic summaries or surveys of data' (Sandelowski and Barroso, 2007: 17), which can either be the final product or be the initial stage before meta-synthesis • Meta-synthesis is 'an interpretive integration of qualitative findings that are themselves interpretive syntheses of data' (Sandelowski and Barroso, 2007: 18)	Bressan, V., Cadorin, L., Stevanin, S. and Palese, A. (2019) 'Patients' experiences of bedside handover: findings from a meta-synthesis', *Scandinavian Journal of Caring Sciences*, 33(3): 556-68.

least two categories (Lockwood et al., 2015). A synthesised finding is the over-arching description of a group of categories. Just as with other systematic reviews, it is expected that the reviewers will explain the processes they undertook not only to identify the findings but also how the categories were developed.

JBI describe meta-aggregation as being in direct contrast to the interpretive approach of meta-ethnography and that it represents 'a goodness of fit with systematic review that is much closer than many other qualitative approaches to synthesis' (Lockwood et al., 2020). However, there have been criticisms of meta-aggregation in that by imitating the processes of a quantitative systematic review, it is trying to over-simplify the complexities of qualitative research and that this will 'inevitably do an injustice to the original studies and fail to advance knowledge in the direction that qualitative investigators envision' (Bergdahl, 2019: 2).

Conclude and make recommendations

The reviewers should justify their conclusions and recommendations in relation both to their application to practice and the implications for healthcare. Recommendations in terms of future research agendas are normally included. Other information such as costs involved in treatment regimes should be addressed.

CRITIQUING A SYSTEMATIC REVIEW

Although the process of undertaking systematic reviews is rigorous, this does not mean that they do not need to be critically appraised. As identified in Chapters 6 and 7, there are a number of tools available to help you undertake critical appraisal (Appendix 3 provides a generic approach to critically appraising systematic reviews). When critically appraising, it may be helpful to have some research books to hand so that information can be checked or clarified. A number of recommended titles are listed at the end of this chapter.

> Identify alternative tools/checklists for critically appraising systematic reviews.
>
> **Activity 8.5**

Applicability to practice

The criteria identified in Chapter 5 for judging applicability to practice are equally valid for systematic reviews; however, there is also another aspect that should be considered. The specificity of a systematic review question means that a very focused aspect of care is usually being considered and there is a clear need to place this within the context of the care environment in question. Consideration also needs to be given as to whether factors not considered in the review will have implications for applying the results to an area of practice.

> Identify a systematic review specific to your area of practice and critically appraise it using the checklist in Appendix 6.
>
> **Activity 8.6**

Summary

- Systematic reviews provide a rigorous review of research findings in relation to a specific question and as such they are fundamental to EBP, providing nurses and other healthcare professionals with sound evidence on which to base practice.

(Continued)

- The systematic review process involves the 'pooling' of results from 'like' studies and creating a larger data set for analysis. This is known as meta-analysis in relation to quantitative research.
- If there is significant heterogeneity within the studies reviewed in a systematic review it is unlikely that the results of the study will be subjected to meta-analysis.
- There are a variety of approaches to the synthesis of qualitative evidence; it is important that a clear description of the approach is provided to allow decisions to be made as to the rigour of the review.

FURTHER READING

Boland, A., Cherry, M.G. and Dixon, R. (eds) (2017) *Doing a Systematic Review: A Student's Guide* (2nd edn). London: Sage.

Gerrish, K. and Lathlean, J. (2015) *The Research Process in Nursing* (7th edn). Oxford: Wiley-Blackwell.

Gough, D., Oliver, S. and Thomas, J. (2017) *An Introduction to Systematic Reviews* (2nd edn). London: Sage.

Holly, C., Salmond, S. and Saimbert, S. (2022) *Comprehensive Systematic Review for Advanced Practice Nursing* (3rd edn). New York: Springer.

Khan, K., Kunz, R., Kleijnen, J. and Antes, G. (2011) *Systematic Reviews to Support Evidence-based Medicine: How to Review and Apply Findings of Healthcare Research* (2nd edn). Boca Raton, FL: CRC Press.

Moule, P., Aveyard, H. and Goodman, M. (2017) *Nursing Research: An Introduction* (3rd edn). London: Sage.

Parahoo, K. (2014) *Nursing Research: Principles, Process and Issues* (3rd edn). Basingstoke: Palgrave Macmillan.

Petticrew, M. and Roberts, H. (2006) *Systematic Reviews in the Social Sciences: A Practical Guide.* Malden, MA: Blackwell Publishing.

Polit, D.F. and Beck, C.T. (2020) *Essentials of Nursing Research: Appraising Evidence for Nursing Practice* (10th edn). Philadelphia: Wolters Kluwer Health.

USEFUL WEBLINKS

Campbell Collaboration: an international social science research network that produces systematic reviews and other evidence syntheses in relation to crime and justice, disability, education, international development and social welfare. These are published in the open access journal *Campbell Systematic Reviews*.

www.campbellcollaboration.org

https://onlinelibrary.wiley.com/journal/18911803

Centre for Reviews and Dissemination: provides guidance on conducting systematic reviews. They also produce PROSPERO, an international register of prospectively registered systematic reviews in health and social care.

CRD Guidance: www.york.ac.uk/crd/guidance

PROSPERO: www.crd.york.ac.uk/PROSPERO

Cochrane Library: includes the Cochrane Database of Systematic Reviews, which is the leading resource for systematic reviews in healthcare: www.cochranelibrary.com

EPPI-Centre: undertakes, supports and develops methods for systematic reviews and synthesis of research evidence. Their knowledge library provides a browsable list of systematic reviews in a wide range of fields including education, health promotion and public health: https://eppi.ioe.ac.uk/cms

JBI Evidence Synthesis: an international, peer-reviewed online journal that publishes systematic and scoping reviews (and protocols): https://journals.lww.com/jbisrir

Conclusion to Part II

The aim of Part II was to provide you with the necessary skills, knowledge and tools to enable you to critically appraise a range of evidence. Hopefully you have now:

- identified a number of papers relevant to your own area of practice;
- found a number of appropriate tools to aid you in your critical appraisal;
- identified gaps in your knowledge and developed action plans to allow you to fill in the gaps;
- developed confidence in your ability to critically appraise evidence in an appropriate way.

Part II ends with a word search puzzle in which there are 21 words associated with Chapters 5, 6, 7 and 8. What are they? The answers can be found on p. 219.

J	T	R	I	A	L	U	O	U	T	Q	T	V	Q	U	X	T	E	V	X
A	G	M	U	Q	V	A	R	I	A	B	L	E	S	E	L	R	O	E	D
S	K	S	Q	Q	L	X	R	I	G	O	U	R	E	B	H	U	M	G	H
K	V	S	J	R	S	J	C	F	D	N	B	T	Y	T	N	S	N	Z	S
K	W	Y	B	F	N	K	O	Q	A	P	F	B	E	R	Z	T	J	R	T
M	A	Z	R	T	O	Q	N	N	Z	R	E	J	U	A	Z	W	D	A	R
O	V	H	A	T	W	E	F	Z	R	O	Z	F	I	N	Y	O	E	N	A
D	S	Y	C	D	B	Y	I	X	E	B	U	F	J	S	H	R	P	D	T
E	M	P	K	W	A	R	R	K	L	A	P	E	Q	F	F	T	E	O	I
R	E	O	E	A	L	E	M	E	I	B	T	T	L	E	F	H	N	M	F
Y	T	T	T	J	L	D	A	F	A	I	K	I	A	R	E	I	D	I	I
A	A	H	I	L	R	V	B	X	B	L	D	C	L	A	W	N	A	S	E
K	A	E	N	D	E	O	I	G	I	I	G	D	N	B	Z	E	B	E	D
E	N	S	G	I	Q	B	L	E	L	T	U	U	L	I	W	S	I	D	S
U	A	I	T	U	R	K	I	E	I	Y	F	G	K	L	Z	S	L	O	S
N	L	S	T	V	P	B	T	Z	T	F	F	Z	U	I	V	E	I	A	B
K	Y	C	W	R	W	J	Y	A	Y	M	E	A	N	T	K	R	T	C	P
L	S	U	J	E	M	I	C	B	A	S	N	K	M	Y	V	W	Y	G	O
S	I	U	F	R	T	Z	Y	P	R	I	V	A	L	I	D	I	T	Y	T
C	S	K	C	R	E	D	I	B	I	L	I	T	Y	T	D	F	R	C	B

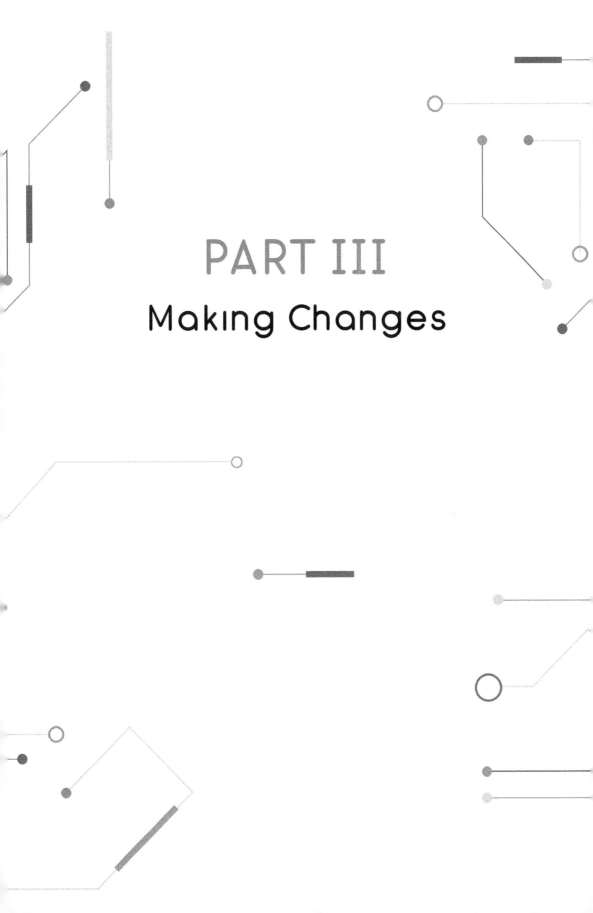

PART III
Making Changes

9

Evaluation, Audit and Research

Paul Linsley

Learning Outcomes

By the end of the chapter, you will be able to:

- define the terms evaluation, audit and research;
- discuss the key features and differences of each;
- discuss various approaches and challenges associated with conducting evaluation research;
- consider stakeholder involvement when conducting an evaluation;
- understand what is meant by theory driven evaluation.

INTRODUCTION

The following chapter looks at the difference between service evaluation, audit and research. Put simply, nursing research involves finding the answers to questions about 'what nurses should do to help patients', audit examines 'whether nurses are doing this, and if not, why not', and service evaluation asks about 'the effect of nursing care on patient experiences and outcomes' (Wade, 2005: 486). Whilst there are differences between the three there are also some similarities, and each can be considered evidence. All three involve the collection and presentation of data and are used to shape clinical practice. Whilst there are distinct differences between the three, they can become blurred and their use problematic especially when meeting governance and approval requirements such as ethics. Knowing the difference between health service evaluation, audit and research can be tricky especially for the clinician in practice. Each area of interest will be explored in greater depth and their use as part of evidence-based practice highlighted. The chapter also looks at theory-driven evaluation as a research methodology and focuses on the use and development of Realistic Evaluation, which is gaining popularity as a research methodology for exploring health and social care practice.

RESEARCH

Research has been defined as 'the attempt to derive generalisable or transferable new knowledge to answer or refine relevant questions with scientifically sound methods. It includes activities that are carried out in preparation for or as a consequence of the interventional part of the research, such as screening potential participants for eligibility, obtaining participants' consent and publishing results' (National Institute for Health Research, 2018). It also includes 'non-interventional health and social care research (i.e. projects that do not involve any change in standard treatment, care or other services), projects that aim to generate hypotheses, methodological research and descriptive research' (Health Research Authority, 2017: 6). By definition, this excludes audits or practice and service evaluations. It also excludes needs assessments, quality improvement, routine banking of biological samples or data except where this activity is integral to a self-contained research project designed to test a clear hypothesis. Research seeks to create new knowledge and understanding through logical reasoning and is analytical in its exploration and interpretation of data and findings. Research is purposeful when it says something about practice and each study creates a path for generating new questions and in this way moves our understanding of the topic forward.

AUDIT

While research is concerned with discovering the right thing to do, audit is concerned with ensuring that the right thing is done (Smith, 1992). Clinical audit has been described as 'a quality improvement process that seeks to improve patient care and outcomes through systematic review of care against explicit criteria and the implementation of change' (NICE, 2002: 1). Like research, audit 'involves systematically looking at the procedures used for diagnosis, care and treatment, examining how associated resources are used and investigating the effect care has on the outcome and quality of life for the patient' (Twycross and Shorten, 2014: 65). Monitoring progress is a key function to improving services (Social Care Institute for Excellence, 2019). Standards should be based on best practice, which in turn, should be based on best evidence. Research informs standards that audit is to monitor. In common with research the aim of clinical audit is to improve patient outcomes. It measures current practice against evidence-based clinical standards and whether an activity or service is meeting these. This information is usually shared with stakeholders and used as a quality indicator as to how a service is performing. Where a service or team is not meeting a standard, changes can be made at an individual, team or service level to bring the service up to the required standard. Further monitoring undertaken as a re-audit is used to confirm that this has led to an improvement or whether further changes need to be made. Key characteristics of audit activity are outlined in Box 9.1 below.

> ## Box 9.1 Some characteristics of audits
>
> - Clinical audit forms one area of quality assurance.
> - An audit assesses care currently being provided against a predetermined standard (e.g. of performance or clinical benefit).
> - An audit aims to determine if improvements or changes to the current level of service provided are required.
> - An audit may involve service users, carers or staff input.
> - An audit does not carry out any experiments or new treatments/interventions on users.
> - An audit never involves disturbance to users beyond normal clinical management/ practice.
> - No randomisation is involved; and an audit does not require ethical approval.
> - An audit has potential to influence changes in practice.

THE AUDIT CYCLE

Clinical audit should be seen as a continuous cycle of deciding which topics to audit and why; measuring care against standards based on best evidence; acting on findings by making improvements and changes as necessary in line with findings; and sustaining improvements by putting in place measures to maintain standards and re-audit where necessary (Healthcare Quality Improvement Partnership, 2017).

Within the cycle an issue or problem is identified, criteria and standards are set, and data is collected to measure actual performance. See Appendix 7 for a tool to help with action planning. This is then compared to the criteria and standards. If any differences are noted an action plan is created to facilitate changes in practice. Most importantly, once the changes have been implemented the cycle begins again with a re-audit to measure the improvements (see Figure 9.1).

> Take time to look at the type of audits carried out in your workplace. Of each audit, ask: why was the audit needed; on what evidence was the audit based; what evidence is being gathered; and has it led to any changes in clinical practice?
>
> **Activity 9.1**

SERVICE EVALUATION

Service evaluation aims to evaluate the effectiveness or efficiency of a service, with the aim of generating information to inform local decision making (Backhouse and Ogunlayi, 2020). A service evaluation should be 'a rigorous and structured assessment of a completed

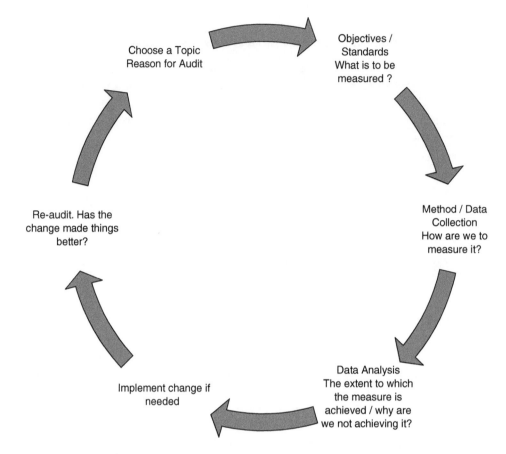

Figure 9.1 The audit cycle

or ongoing activity, intervention, programme or policy that will determine the extent to which it is achieving its objectives and contributing to decision-making' (Menon et al., 2009: 8). Service valuations are designed to answer the question 'what standard does this service achieve?' Whereas audits are designed to find out 'whether the quality of a service meets a defined standard'. In this way, service evaluation provides practical information on which to base decisions as to the worth or value of a service and whether a development or service should be continued or not. As such, it is usually only relevant to the population or setting in which it takes place and results are not generalisable. Service evaluation is not considered research as it does not seek to create new knowledge but to confirm what is known or desired.

Some characteristics of service evaluations:

- Service evaluations define and judge existing service delivery, where research may trial a new approach.
- In service evaluations, agreed levels of service are systematically monitored and evaluated.
- Service evaluations provide practical information such as costs, benefits, strengths and weaknesses of a service.

- Service evaluation determines the value of a service.
- In service evaluations, participants are usually patients/service users, carers or staff.
- Service evaluations do not require ethical approval.
- Service evaluations can use a number of qualitative and/or quantitative research methods.
- Service evaluations provide a 'snapshot' of a service.
- The data collected during an evaluation can be used at a later date for research providing it meets ethical standards.

A service is considered effective if it delivers outputs in accordance with its objectives and is considered efficient or cost-effective if effectiveness is achieved at the lowest practical cost.

The key differences between research, audit and service evaluation described above are summarised in Table 9.1 below.

Table 9.1   Differentiating audit, service evaluation and research

Research	Clinical audit	Service evaluation
The attempt to derive generalisable new knowledge including studies that aim to generate hypotheses as well as studies that aim to test them.	Designed and conducted to produce information to inform delivery of best care.	Designed and conducted solely to define or judge current care.
Quantitative research – designed to test a hypothesis.	Designed to answer the question:	Designed to answer the question:
Qualitative research – identifies/explores themes following established methodology.	'Does this service reach a predetermined standard?'	'What standard does this service achieve?'
Addresses clearly defined questions, aims and objectives.	Measures against a standard.	Measures current service without reference to a standard.
Quantitative research – may involve evaluating or comparing interventions, particularly new ones. Qualitative research – usually involves studying how interventions and relationships. are experienced.	Involves an intervention in use ONLY. (The choice of treatment is that of the clinician and patient according to guidance, professional standards and/or patient preference.)	Involves an intervention in use ONLY. (The choice of treatment is that of the clinician and patient according to guidance, professional standards and/or patient preference.)
Usually involves collecting data that are additional to those for routine care but may include data collected routinely. May involve treatments, samples or investigations additional to routine care.	Usually involves analysis of existing data but may include administration of simple interview or questionnaire.	Usually involves analysis of existing data but may include administration of simple interview or questionnaire.

(Continued)

Table 9.1   (Continued)

Research	Clinical audit	Service evaluation
Quantitative research - study design may involve allocating patients to intervention groups. Qualitative research uses a clearly defined sampling framework underpinned by conceptual or theoretical justifications.	No allocation to intervention groups: the healthcare professional and patient have chosen intervention before clinical audit.	No allocation to intervention groups: the healthcare professional and patient have chosen intervention before service evaluation.
May involve randomisation	No randomisation	No randomisation

Although any of these three may raise ethical issues, under current UK guidance it is only research that requires ethical approval. However, it is suggested that when conducting an audit, service evaluation or research, it should first be discussed with, and approval gained, from your organisation's Research and Development Department.

Source: Defining Research (Health Research Authority, 2009).

Activity 9.2

Look for a service evaluation undertaken of your service. Just as in Activity 9.1, ask: why was the evaluation needed; on what evidence was this based; how was it conducted; and has it led to any changes in clinical practice or the way we do things?

EVALUATION

In its broadest sense, evaluation of any kind is a systematic process to understand what a programme does and how well the programme does it. Evaluation is said to be useful when it provides feedback that can be understood and used by a variety of audiences, including staff, managers, client-groups and other interested parties; often in regard to whether a programme has achieved its intended goals or not. Evaluation can focus on:

Projects: these normally consist of a set of activities undertaken to achieve specific objectives within a given budget and time period.

Programmes: are organised sets of projects or services concerned with a particular sector or geographic region.

Services: are based on a permanent structure, and have the goal of becoming national in coverage, e.g. health services, whereas programmes are usually limited in time or area.

Processes: are organisational operations of a continuous and supporting nature (e.g. personnel procedures, health and safety measures, clinical reporting systems, management operating systems, processes for making referrals).

Conditions: are particular characteristics or states of being of persons or things (e.g. disease, nutritional status, literacy, income level).

(Salama, 2010)

When thinking of a programme as a whole, it is common to break the above process down into three distinct parts: inputs, processes, outputs. Inputs are the resources provided for an activity and include cash, supplies, personnel, equipment and training. Processes are the means by which the programme transforms inputs into outputs. Whereas outputs are the specific products or services that an activity is expected to deliver as a result of receiving the inputs. Traditionally, evaluation is conducted in assessing one of four areas: (1) formative evaluation; (2) process evaluation; (3) outcome evaluation; (4) impact evaluation (see Table 9.2).

1. *Formative evaluation* is usually done at the start of a programme or activity and is used to judge the feasibility, appropriateness and acceptability of the activity before it is fully implemented. It is usually conducted when a new programme is being developed or where an existing one is being adopted or modified.
2. *Process evaluation*, sometimes known as implementation evaluation, is used to determine whether the programme activities have been implemented as intended and the process which was put in place is effective and operating as it should be. This type of evaluation normally consists of a set of activities undertaken to achieve specific objectives within a given budget and time period.
3. *Outcome*, sometimes referred to as effectiveness evaluation, measures the extent to which a programme has met its objectives. Or in terms of an intervention, how effective an intervention has been.
4. *Impact evaluation* provides information about the impacts produced by a programme or intervention, either positive or negative, intended or unintended, direct or indirect.

Planning, implementation and evaluation are all essential components of all programmes. Planning and implementation stages of any programme are vital for ensuring successful outcomes. The planning and implementation phases of programmes, however, are only part of the process, therefore should always be monitored and followed up by an evaluation phase. Not to do this would in most cases invalidate what's gone previously, as well as provide no real means with which to measure the validity or success of a programme. It is rare to see evidence of an evaluations process at the start of programmes and they are usually served as an add on, often when the programme or activity is near to completion.

While assessing the outcomes of a service or intervention is important, outcomes mean different things to different people. If a service has specified goals or objectives, then an obvious outcome is to assess whether these have been achieved. A serious shortcoming of this tight objectives-linked approach is that services and interventions involving people are notorious for having unanticipated consequences (either in addition to, or instead of, the proposed ones). Increasingly, researchers and staff are using different approaches to evaluation; while many of these maintain an element of outcome evaluation, they seek to evaluate other elements of the programme or intervention.

Properly conducted evaluation can help services to meet needs of users and can identify areas which need improvement. Evaluation can also be used in the design of services, to assess how well the services are working, and to find out whether services are effective. It can also be used to help support the case for funding. Showing that services work well can help attract further support. Another important point to remember about evaluating programmes is that it allows practitioners to design and implement new ones. They can learn from the strengths and weaknesses of previous programmes and build on these.

Table 9.2   Different types of evaluation and when you might use them

Evaluation types	When to use	What it shows	Why its useful
Formative evaluation	During the development of a new programme When an existing programme is being modified or is being used in a new setting or with a new population To target a new problem or behaviour	Whether the proposed programme elements are likely to be needed, understood and accepted by the population you want to reach The extent to which an evaluation is possible, based on the goals and objectives	It allows for modifications to be made to the plan before full implementation begins Maximises the likelihood that the programme will succeed If a programme is in operation, but having unanticipated problems, a formative evaluation may help find the cause
Process evaluation	As soon as programme implementation begins During operation of an existing programme	How well the programme is working The extent to which the programme is being implemented as designed Whether the programme is accessible and acceptable to its target population	Provides an early warning for any problems that may occur Allows programmes to monitor how well their programme plans and activities are working Can provide encouragement to participants
Outcome evaluation Objectives-based evaluation	After the programme has made contact with at least one person or group in the target population	The degree to which the programme is having an effect on the target population's behaviour	Tells whether the programme is being effective in meeting its objectives Results can be used to justify continuation of the programme or activity or intervention
Impact evaluation	During the operation of an existing programme at appropriate intervals At the end of a programme	The degree to which the programme meets its ultimate goal	Provides evidence for use in policy and funding decisions Allows programmes to learn from their successes and failures and to incorporate what they have learnt into their current or next project Provides evidence of success for use in future requests for funding

(Adapted from: *W.K. Kellogg Foundation Evaluation Handbook 2001* and Department of Health and Human Resources USA, 2018)

STAKEHOLDER INVOLVEMENT

Whilst Guba and Lincoln (1989: 21), leading writers on evaluation, argued that 'there was no right way to define evaluation', they were critical of the commitment to the scientific paradigm of enquiry, and the tendency towards 'managerialism' in evaluative studies. By 'managerialism' they meant the situation in which the 'manager' commissioner, of an evaluation, or sponsor stands outside of the process and, therefore, if a failure in the programme is identified, other personnel are blamed. Since the manager also decides the extent to which the results will be published, Guba and Lincoln (1989) argued that stakeholders, or those affected by the evaluation results, will be disempowered. So, a lack of attention to the questions of whose values would dominate an evaluation and how value differences can be negotiated, becomes a problem to be addressed as part of any evaluation.

Wye and McClenaghan (2000) identified four factors when putting evidence into practice:

1. Resources need to be sufficient.
2. **The proposed change needs to offer benefits of real interest to staff who have to change.**
3. **Enough of the right people need to be on board early enough.**
4. The approach needs to be interactive and relate research to current practice.

Two of these four factors, highlighted in bold, are explicitly about stakeholders – the other two are implicitly about stakeholders. In order to ensure that enough of the right people are on board early enough we need to identify these people at an early point in the process.

Spend a few minutes considering who stakeholders are, what they are and what we mean by stakeholders. An example answer is given at the end of the chapter.

Activity 9.3

To help us identify such stakeholders we could consider:

- Who will be affected by the change?
- Will it impact other care settings?
- Who has the power to make the change?
- Who will be affected by the change?
- Will it impact other care settings?
- Who has the power to make the change?
- Who are potential allies?
- Who are potential opponents?

- Who are the minority/rarely heard voices?
- Who can contribute or block resources needed?
- And who will be responsible for managing the outcome?

(After Reed et al., 2017)

It is important to remember that not all stakeholders are equal. They can have more or less power in relation to your proposed change, but at the same time they can also have more or less interest in your proposed change. So, at one extreme you can have a highly powerful stakeholder who has no interest in your proposed change, or a less powerful stakeholder who is highly interested in your proposed change. What you really want, of course, is a highly powerful stakeholder who is highly interested in your proposed change. It is therefore useful to map who are the stakeholders when planning an evaluation. This is useful as it can help you identify and develop strategies for managing them and to assess the feasibility of the project. What we are trying to achieve in stakeholder mapping is not just who is involved, but why they are involved, what each stakeholder's agenda is, and what their potential input to change might be. And that input might be positive or negative. As Greenhalgh (2017) put it:

> People are not passive recipients of innovations. Rather (and to a greater or lesser extent in different individuals), they seek innovations out, experiment with them, evaluate them, find (or fail to find) meaning in them, develop feelings (positive or negative) about them, challenge them, worry about them, complain about them, 'work round' them, talk to others about them, develop know-how about them, modify them to fit particular tasks, and attempt to improve or redesign them (often through dialogue with other users).

WHEN IS EVALUATION RESEARCH?

Evaluation research is recognised as a research approach in its own right. It is used extensively in both health and education to maintain and improve the quality of programmes. In its broadest sense, evaluation is a systematic process to understand what the programme does and how well the programme does it. Furthermore, it is the examination of events and conditions that have (or are presumed to have) occurred at an earlier time, or are unfolding as the evaluation takes place. In order to do this, these events and conditions must exist, must be describable, must have occurred or be occurring. Evaluation then is retrospective in that the emphasis is on what has been or is being observed, not what is likely to happen (Rossi et al., 2004).

Like any other form of research, evaluative research is a process of systematic enquiry that entails collection of data; documentation of critical information; and analysis and interpretation of the data/information, in accordance with suitable methodologies set by specific professional fields and academic disciplines. Evaluation research is a type of applied research, and so it is intended to have some real-world effect. Many methods like surveys and experiments can be used to do evaluation research. The process of evaluation research consisting of data analysis and reporting is a rigorous, systematic process that involves collecting data about organisations, processes, projects, services and/or resources. Evaluation research enhances knowledge and decision making, and leads to practical applications. When putting together any evaluative research study, the following should be given due consideration.

Scope of the evaluation

- goals and objectives;
- conceptual framework correlating inputs, processes, outputs and outcomes;
- identification of stakeholders;
- ethical issues.

Methodological approach

- study design;
- data collection and data analysis methods;
- interval between data collection points;
- sample.

Implementation plan

- selection of geographic areas;
- roles and responsibilities;
- timetable for identified activities;
- preparation of budget;
- dissemination plan for evaluation results.

THEORY-DRIVEN EVALUATION

We will now look at theory-driven evaluation, an increasingly popular form of evaluative research, and in particular Realistic Evaluation (Pawson and Tilley, 1997). Theory-driven evaluation is considered an approach in its own right and seeks to create new knowledge. Theory-driven evaluation is defined as the systematic application of social research procedures in assessing conceptualisation and design, implementation, and utility of social intervention programmes (Rossi and Freeman, 1985). It provides a contextual or holistic assessment of a programme and is used for prescribing evaluation purposes, general activities, strategies and methods in the form of a 'programme theory' (Derbyshire, 2018).

Theory-driven evaluation involves the construction of a detailed programme theory that is then used to guide the evaluation (Alkin and Christie, 2004). It guides the design and conduct of an evaluation study in terms of delimiting the target population who would benefit from the services offered by the programme, developing procedures that guide the programme operations and monitoring, and selecting the concepts and variables to be measured and the timing or occasions of their measurement (Shadish et al., 1991).

Key elements of a theory-based evaluation (White, 2009) include the following:

- It is designed to answer the question of what worked (by measuring or assessing the changes brought about by a development intervention), but also why and how it worked (by examining the processes that led to those changes).
- It generally examines wider contributions to change, such as the actions of other interventions or changes in the wider socioeconomic environment.
- It works with an explicit theory – e.g. a theory of change or logic model – that under-pins the development intervention being evaluated.
- It is based on two distinct parts: a conceptual part, which concentrates on developing the theory of change or logic model and using it to guide the evaluation; and a second part that involves collecting evidence to establish whether and/or how an intervention produced the desired changes.

In general, a theory-based evaluation always consists of three major components:

- the use, adaptation or development of a theory of change or logic model to explicitly set out the theory of the intervention;
- the collection of information at different levels of the theory to see whether or not, or how far, the desired changes have occurred; and
- an exploration of the links between changes at the different levels to test assumptions, and to confirm or reject the theory linking the levels.

Chen and Rossi (1981) advocated theory-driven evaluation which seeks to identify how or why a programme outcome is achieved. Theory-driven evaluation has been created in many different ways and used for a number of purposes. In some evaluations, the pro-gramme theory has been developed largely by the evaluator, based on a review of the literature on similar programmes; through discussions with key informants, or through the observations of the programme itself. In other evaluations, the programme theory is being developed primarily by those associated with the programme, often through a group process. Many practitioners advise using a combination of these approaches. Within this diversity, it is possible to identify two broad clusters of practice. In some programme theory evaluations, the main purpose of the evaluation is to test the programme theory, to identify what it is about the programme that causes the outcomes. This sort of programme theory evaluation is most commonly used in large, well-resourced evaluations focused on such questions as, does this programme work? Or should this pilot be extended? These theory-testing evaluations wrestle with the issue of causal attributions – sometimes using experimental or quasi-experimental designs in conjunction with programme theory and sometimes using programme theory as an alternative to these designs. Such evaluations can be particularly helpful in distinguishing between theory failure and implementation failure.

The other type of programme evaluation is often seen in small-scale evaluations done at the project level by or on behalf of project managers and staff. In these cases, programme theory is more likely to be used for formative evaluation, to guide their daily actions and decisions rather than for summative evaluation. Such programme theories are often not concerned with causal attribution. Although this type of programme does not show the relationship among different components, these relationships are sometimes explored in the empirical component of the evaluation. Whilst some of these evaluations pay attention to the influence of external factors, there is rarely systematic ruling out of rival explanations for the outcomes. Many of these evaluations have been developed in response to the increasing demands for programmes and agencies to report performance information and to demonstrate their use of evaluation to improve services. In these circumstances, programme theory has often been highly regarded because of the benefits it provides to programme managers and staff in terms of improved planning and management, in addition to its use as an evaluation tool.

Theory-driven evaluation appears under a number of different headings, including pro-gramme theory evaluation (see Chen, 1990), theory of action, theory of change (see Weiss, 1995, 2000), programme logic, logical frameworks (see Kaplan and Garrett, 2005), and realist or realistic evaluation (Pawson and Tilley, 1997). It is the latter, realistic evaluation that we will now focus on.

REALISTIC EVALUATION

The use of realistic evaluation (Pawson and Tilley, 1997) by nurse researchers has gained in popularity over the last several years. Realistic evaluation is a form of theory-driven evaluation derived from, and founded on, the work of philosopher Roy Bhaskar and his writings on Critical Realism (1975).

The critical part of critical realism reflects a critical social science view, namely that social science should be critical of the practices it studies (Sayer, 2000: 173) and holds similarities with a Marxist view that what is apparent on the surface is often masking an underlying reality. As part of evaluation critical realism places an importance on the social world in which people move, and that to understand the behaviour, values and meanings of any given individual (or group), account must be made of the culture in which they operate. The objective then is to display the social organisation of activities, as they are revealed through involvement in the natural setting of the activity. The researcher's atten-tion is directed towards participants' subjective perceptions of their own experiences with the aim of presenting these perceptions clearly and understanding their basic structure and meaning through a process of interpretation. Realism therefore explores the assumptions on which practices are based, not only uncovering false knowledge and beliefs, but provid-ing explanations as to why these beliefs are held. This is a particularly relevant consideration within health as inequities are continuing to widen, despite our awareness of their exist-ence (Wilson and Greenhill, 2000). The critical realist tries to make sense of what people are doing by asking 'What's going on here? How does this work? How do people do this?' And hopes to be told by people about 'the way we do things around here' (Pawson and Tilley, 1997). To this end, realistic evaluation does not attempt to verify pre-existing theory; rather it focuses on the discovery of theory.

Wilson and Greenhill (2004) have suggested critical realism works in this way through four modes: questioning the status quo, challenging ideology, focus on equality and ine-quality, and commitment to emancipation. Let us take the example of health inequalities. Increasingly, health issues such as obesity, diabetes and other long-term conditions are attributed to avoidable factors such as lifestyle choices and health behaviours, and concerns over the sustainability of a universal healthcare system gives rise to debates about where the responsibility for health should lie. This necessitates consideration of the ways in which societal and systemic factors impinge on health decisions, and those individual actions are rooted in societal contexts. Through studying the real social forces which constrain human action and studying social structures and agency as separate but interrelated entities, it is possible to not only understand the way things are, but how the current state of affairs has emerged (Behari-Leak, 2017). The realist view of complexity acknowledges the inter-dependency on the part of individuals, healthcare systems and society in tackling health inequalities (Scambler, 2018).

A key premise to critical realism is that the concepts of truth and falsity do not provide a coherent view of the relationship between knowledge and object. Rather, knowledge is the social and historical product. Mancias and Secord (1983) emphasised the complexity of the real world, where more complex layers of reality can be found to explain other levels. This means participants' actions will be embedded within an organisation, for example, of the National Health Service, the hospital or community, as well as their own personal experiences of healthcare. Indeed, Pawson and Tilley (1997: 36) contended that:

A programme is its personnel, its place, its past and its prospects.

By studying social phenomena within the context of realistic methodology the emphasis is on coming to terms with the meaning and experience of those being studied within their natural circumstances; that is, the sense, and the experiences, participants use to construct, maintain and negotiate courses of social action. The implications of this position are far reaching. The accounts that participants give to their actions are indexed to particular situations (i.e. time, space, place, etc.), and though similarities may exist between each other's accounts, they tend to conceal complex, local-specific meanings. Second, the application of social rules (i.e. acceptable behaviour within a given situation) requires individuals to make judgements about meanings (i.e. social etiquette and engagement). However, indexicalibility inhibits gen-eralisations because there are no privileged accounts, outside the situated accounts. Instead, rules are resources upon which people routinely draw in the situated nature of their activities.

Bhaskar states that realism has a 'Real emancipatory impulse' (1989: 169). Emancipation requires change, and realism sees the potential for change in unexercised causal powers; 'our descriptions do not exhaust possibilities' (Bhaskar, 1989: 170), thus there are many possibil-ities of how things could be different. Considering these issues also calls for a consideration of the ethical issues this gives rise to. Whilst criticising bad practices displays an assump-tion that there is a better alternative, what is more difficult to establish is what should be deemed as better. As Sayer (2011: 223) states, 'It is one thing to argue that all people are of equal worth, quite another that their ideas are too.' Critical social science demands a reflexive exploration of values, standpoints and normative theory.

Pawson and Tilley (1997: 71) described the logic of realist evaluation as follows:

The basic task of social inquiry is to explain interesting, puzzling, socially significant regularities. Realism views regularities in a loose sense, acknowledging the possibil-ities of what might actually happen can be dependent on a number of different mechanisms interacting, thus regularities within an open system are never certain, as opposed to those observed in controlled experiments, and have thus been termed demi-regularities which display a tendency rather than a law of science, for which the value is explanatory rather than predicative. In Realism explanation takes the form of posting some underlying mechanism, which generates the demi regularity and thus consists of propositions about how the interplay between structure and agency has constituted the regularity. Within realist investigation there is also investigation of how the working of such mechanisms are contingent and conditional, and thus only fired in particular local, historical or institutional contexts.

Broadly speaking, realistic evaluation focuses on understanding and explaining how programmes work, for whom and in what circumstances (Pawson and Tilley, 1997: 220).

Realistic evaluation stresses four key linked concepts for explaining and understanding programmes (Pawson and Tilley, 1997: 222): 'mechanism', 'context', 'outcome pattern' and 'context-mechanism-outcome pattern configuration'.

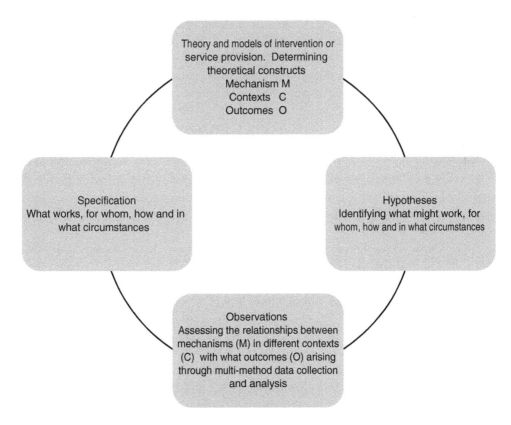

Figure 9.2 The realistic evaluation cycle

(Adapted from Pawson and Tilley, 1997; Kazi et al., 2002)

A CMO configuration is a proposition stating what it is about an initiative that works for whom in what circumstances. This process of how subjects interpret and act upon an intervention stratagem is known as the programme mechanism, and it is the pivot around which realist research revolves. The metaphor of the mechanism is useful to explain how a programme may or may not work. The step is taken from asking whether a programme works, to what it is about the circumstances of the programme that makes it work. By works, it is meant the beneficial impact on the participants of the individual programmes. It would be insufficient to suggest a programme works just because of its introduction into a clinical area.

Identifying the crucial programme mechanisms is only the first step in a realist evaluation. It is also always assumed that they will be active only under particular circumstances, that is, contexts. Contexts describe those features of the conditions in which programmes are introduced that are relevant to the operation of the programme mechanisms. Realism utilises contextual thinking to address the issues of 'for whom' and 'in what circumstances' a programme will work.

Programmes are almost always introduced into multiple contexts, in the sense that mechanisms activated by the interventions will vary and will do so according to saliently different conditions. Because of relevant variations in contexts and mechanisms thereby activated, any programme is liable to have mixed outcome patterns. Outcome patterns comprise the intended and unintended consequences of programmes, resulting from the activation of different contexts. Realism does not rely on a single outcomes measure to deliver a pass/fail verdict on a programme. Nor does it make a hard and fast distinction between outputs (intermediate implementation targets) and outcomes (changes in the behaviour targeted). A realistic evaluation researcher is not just inspecting outcomes in order to see if an initiative works, but is analysing the outcomes to discover if the conjectured mechanism/context theories are confirmed.

In this way, effectiveness of the programme is apprehended with an explanation of why the outcomes developed as they did, and how the programme was able to react to the other underlying mechanisms, and in what contexts. This analysis provides not only evidence of effectiveness, but also an explanation that helps to develop and to improve both content and the targeting of future programmes.

Realistic explanation, therefore, is based on the proposition that causal outcomes follow from mechanisms acting in contexts. A realistic evaluation cycle involves framing theories which identify and explain regularities, deriving hypotheses concerning what might work for whom in what circumstances, testing these through multi-method data collection analysis, which can then inform further generalisations and lead to provision of theory and new hypotheses. Thus, we begin by expecting measures to have varying impact depending on the conditions in which they are introduced and actioned.

Theory includes proposition on how the mechanisms introduced by an intervention into a pre-existing context can generate outcomes. This entails theoretical analysis of mechanisms, contexts and expected outcomes. This can be done using logic of analogy and metaphor. The metaphor of the 'mechanism' is used to explain how a programme works, to what it is about the circumstances of the programme that make it work. The second step consists of generating 'hypotheses'. Typically, the following questions would be addressed in the hypotheses: (1) what changes or outcomes will be brought about by the intervention?

(2) what contexts impinge on this? and (3) what mechanisms (social, cultural and others) would enable these changes, and which one might disable the intervention? A mechanism explains what is responsible for the 'regularity' (Pawson and Tilley, 1997: 71) or outcomes found in the results of the study. This relationship between causal mechanisms and their effects is not fixed but contingent (upon the context in which the mechanisms are activated) (Sayer, 2000: 107). As Pawson (2002) has argued, some programmes may work for some people, some of the time. The third step is the selection of appropriate data collection methods. In this step, it might be possible to provide evidence of the intervention's ability to change reality. Based on the results from the third step, we may return to the programme (the intervention) to make it more specific as an intervention of practice. Next, but not finally, we return to theory. The theory may be developed, the hypotheses refined, the data collection methods enhanced, etc.

In the critical worldview, programme outcomes cannot be explained in isolation; rather, they can only be explained in the sense of a mechanism that is introduced to effect change in a constellation of other mechanisms and structures, embedded in the context of pre-existing historical, economic, cultural, social and other conditions. In this way, the effectiveness of the programme is apprehended with an explanation of why the outcomes developed as they did, and how the programme was able to react to the other underlying mechanisms, and in what contexts. This analysis provides not only evidence of effectiveness, but an explanation that helps to develop and to improve both content and the targeting of future programmes.

Find a realistic evaluation on a topic of your choice. Compare this study with the service evaluation you looked at in Activity 9.2. What are the differences between the two types of evaluation? Did you recognise the realistic evaluation study as research?

Activity 9.4

Summary

- There are distinct differences between research, audit and service evaluation, which can be difficult for clinicians to understand.
- Research involves finding the answers to questions about 'what nurses should do to help patients'; audit examines 'whether nurses are doing this, and if not, why not'; and service evaluation asks about 'the effect of nursing care on patient experiences and outcomes'.
- Despite their differences there are clear similarities between service evaluation, audit and research. All start with important questions, require data to answer the questions, and each needs a systematic approach and sound design.

(Continued)

- Evaluation is recognised as a research approach in its own right when the purpose is to create new knowledge and done with rigour.
- We have seen the emergence of theory-driven evaluation and this is now proving popular in investigating health and social care programmes and interventions. Realistic evaluation is a good example of this and probably the best known of the theory-driven evaluation approaches.
- Properly conducted evaluation can help to tailor services to meet the needs of users and can identify areas which need further improvement.
- The importance of stakeholders' involvement in evaluation and research is highlighted.

FURTHER READING

Brain, J., Schofield, J., Gerrish, K., Mawson, S., Mabbott, I., Dipak, P. and Gerrish, P. (2011) *A Guide for Clinical Audit, Research and Service Review*. Sheffield: Healthcare Quality Improvement Partnership.

Chen, L.-Y.A. and Fawcett, T.N. (2019) 'Service evaluation: A grey area of research?', *Nursing Ethics, 26*(4): 1172–85. doi:10.1177/0969733017742961

USEFUL WEBLINKS

Better Evaluation: a website promoting the use of evaluative research. Many useful resources and information on conducting an evaluative study. www.betterevaluation.org/en/what–evaluation

NHS Evaluation Works: the website includes a toolkit to help with planning and running an evaluative study. And in the resources section it has a number of videos and case studies taking you through the process from start to finish. https://nhsevaluationtoolkit.net/

Answer to Activity 9.3

Stakeholders		
• Influencers	• Referrers	• People
• Adopters	• Providers	• Teams
• Engagers	• Recipients	• Organisations
• Sufferers		• Systems
• Opponents		• Patients
• Challengers		• Families
• Blockers		• Public
• Champions		
• Advocates		

Compare your notes to the table above.

Each of the three columns takes a slightly different approach to identifying other terms we could use to describe stakeholders:

- the first column is about responses to change;
- the second is about existing roles;
- and the third are more organisational categories.

It is suggested that these are useful terms to think about when trying to identify potential stakeholders.

10

Evidence into Practice: Practice Development, Improvement and Innovation

Karen Johnston and Paul Linsley

Learning Outcomes

By the end of the chapter, you will be able to:

- define the terms improvement and innovation;
- discuss the key features of practice development;
- discuss the need for practice innovation;
- identify how to introduce new evidence into the practice setting;
- discuss various approaches and challenges associated with the management of change;
- consider how to develop an evidenced-based culture in the practice setting.

INTRODUCTION

We are living in a fast-moving world where our understanding of what can be achieved in healthcare is constantly being reframed by advances in science and technology and changes to the world in which we live. A major challenge in healthcare is valuing the continual discovery of new knowledge, assessing it for appropriateness for inclusion in care delivery and putting into practice the knowledge that exists. Evidence-based practice, as we have seen, has the power not only to inform but transform practice. Despite this, there remain a number of difficulties getting evidence adopted and integrated into clinical practice. The challenge we face is how to increase the rate of adoption and continue the movement from a profession based on ritual and tradition to using a wide range of evidence.

The transferring of evidence into practice is often a daunting, difficult and complex activity. Simply informing people of the latest research findings does not automatically result in new approaches being adopted and it cannot be assumed that developments in knowledge and skills will result in changes to practice. For instance, most people know that hand washing is central to reducing infections and yet large numbers of health professionals fail to do this appropriately.

Practice development, improvement and innovation are seen as an integral part of today's healthcare system and the answer to modern-day demands. Perhaps the biggest challenge faced by staff today is the need to provide a high standard of care within increasingly limited budgets. Judicial use of the available evidence and research is of great importance when supporting claims of improvement and innovation. It is apparent that EBP has become firmly established in guiding practice-based decisions and interventions and that it represents the key approach for developing and sustaining high-quality, patient-centred care. However, achieving quality improvement and efficiency is a complex activity that requires careful thought and attention. These issues will now be explored and the importance of EBP highlighted when responding to changes in practice.

Before reading the rest of the chapter, consider what the terms practice development, improvement and innovation mean to you. Can you give examples of each based on what you have read in the literature or observed in clinical practice? Compare your observations and comments with what follows.

Activity 10.1

PRACTICE DEVELOPMENT

A wider choice of different types of health services is increasingly becoming available to patients to enable personalised care, faster treatments and personal support through the processes of practice development. A number of definitions have been used to describe practice development; perhaps the best known of these is that put forward by Kitson (1994: 319) who described it as:

> … a system whereby identified or appointed **change agents** work with staff to help them introduce a new activity or practice. The findings may come from the findings of rigorous research; findings of less rigorous research; experience which has not been tested systematically or trying out an idea in practice. The introduction of the development ought to be systematic and carefully evaluated to ensure that the new practice has achieved the improvement intended.

Furthermore, it is:

> … a continuous process of developing person-centred cultures. It is enabled by facilitators who authentically engage with individuals and teams to blend personal qualities and creative imagination with practice skills and practice wisdom. The learning that occurs brings about transformations of individual and team practices. This is sustained by embedding both processes and outcomes in corporate strategy. (Manley et al., 2008: 9)

In this way, practice development plays a pivotal role in fostering a culture and context that nurtures evidence-based practice because it is an:

> … approach that synthesises activities and theory of quality improvement, evidence-base and innovations in practice, within a real-practice context, and with a central focus on the improvement of care and services for patients and clients. (Page and Hammer, 2002: 6)

Practice development covers such activity as quality improvement, practice innovation, the setting and monitoring of standards, and staff development and training. In this way, practice development draws on and synthesises theory and activity from a number of fields and disciplines, such as evidence-based practice, clinical audit, satisfaction surveys, emergent research, and national guidelines issued by professional and government bodies.

Over time, the term practice development has become associated with supporting the modernisation of healthcare and covers a wide range of activities designed to move practice forward in a timely and orderly manner. Healthcare workers as teams of multi-professional practitioners across a range of agencies or settings develop knowledge and skills to influence best practice, experience and outcomes for patients and their families, enhancing organisational and team culture and safety (Dewing et al., 2015). In this way, practice development is collaborative, underpinned by the active engagement of practitioners, and focuses on the improvement of patient care.

In order to develop practice, there is a requirement to not only consider what we are doing, but why we are doing it. Questions to consider might include:

- Do new technologies or new ways of working require new skills and competences?
- Are staff located in organisations within the system in the most meaningful way for the service user?
- What numbers of workforce does the system need to deliver its purpose? Does working as a system create efficiency savings/areas of duplication? Do new ways of working require more people in other roles?
- Does the system have the right balance of clinical to non-clinical roles and managers to frontline workers?
- What are the current finances and how is workforce spend likely to change in the next five years?

PRACTICE IMPROVEMENT

Innovation and improvement are often intertwined in terms of service transformation; however, it is important to distinguish the two. Improvement might be minor changes to a system that works well but may enhance patient experience and satisfaction or reduce waste, waiting times or ensure effective communication. Improvement is designing or redesigning processes and systems to deliver healthcare with improved outcomes and reduced costs. Use of established improvement methodology can be utilised to improve single services or processes or impact on the wider system across organisational boundaries (NHS Leadership Academy, 2016).

In the healthcare context it is necessary to be clear about what we are trying to accomplish. This needs to identify the rationale for improvement but also focus on problems that concern staff or patients. Any change needs to align to national and local delivery targets, plans and frameworks and have clear timescales, costs and data analysis and projections to measure outcomes (NHS England and NHS Improvement, 2019). In order to develop practice, there is a requirement to not only consider what we are doing, but why we are doing it. The model for improvement (Institute for Healthcare Improvement, 2019) asks three questions:

1. What are you trying to achieve?
2. How will you know a change is an improvement?
3. What changes can you make that will result in the improvement that you seek?

Practice improvement also involves examining the way in which a service is run, the way in which staff practise, as well as the way in which patients are treated. The goal of practice improvement is to achieve a higher quality experience for patients (Maher and Panny, 2005). Improvement thinking involves four equally important and interrelated parts that are essential for improvement activities, these being:

- personal and organisational development: building a culture that supports improvement;
- process and systems thinking: understanding work processes and systems, and the linkages within them;
- involving users, carers, staff and the public: understanding their experiences and needs;
- making it a habit: initiating, sustaining and spreading, building improvement into daily work.

(Penny, 2003)

Look at an improvement in your area of interest. What drove this improvement? How did it come about? What evidence underpinned its introduction? How was its impact measured? Did it achieve all its aims?

Activity 10.2

Achieving improvements in clinical practice requires the collaborative effort of the team and all members should feel empowered to contribute. However, this is not always easy to achieve. Healthcare services are seldom static – they evolve over time as the attitudes of those that use the service change with developments in thinking and technology. Some changes are not intentional, while others are desired and required. Increasingly, changes are being made quickly and do not allow for a period of adjustment, which can leave staff feeling powerless and not engaged with. It is important to remember that: 'Not every change is an improvement but certainly every improvement is a change, and we cannot improve something unless we change it' (Goldratt, 1999: 10).

PRACTICE INNOVATION

Innovation comes from the Latin roots of the word, 'in-nova-tion' which means 'restoration' or renewal. Nurses are in an ideal position to change and challenge practice as they provide most of the care delivered worldwide. Innovation involves thinking about new ways of doing things. It requires us to think creatively and flexibly to generate new ideas to solve old problems. Innovation is when a creative idea is put into action, and has been defined as:

> The intentional introduction and application within a role, group, or organisation, of ideas, processes, products or procedures, new to the relevant unit of adoption, designed to significantly benefit the individual, group or wider society. (West, 1990: 16)

This definition captures the three most important characteristics of innovation: (a) novelty, (b) an application component and (c) an intended benefit (Lansisalmi et al., 2006). It implies a real change in the way that things are done and a desire to move practice forward. It requires a commitment to improvement and service development and should be based on sound and demonstrable evidence. Healthcare innovation can be defined as:

> ... the introduction of a new concept, idea, service, process, or product aimed at improving treatment, diagnosis, education, outreach, prevention and research, and with the long-term goals of improving quality, safety, outcomes, efficiency and costs. (Omachonu and Einspruch, 2016)

So, innovation is the introduction of a new way of thinking or working, often including radical change in delivery of services and where they are delivered, as well as adoption and spread to increase impact and reduce unwarranted variation across communities (NHS England, 2016). Practice innovation might include clinical trials, radical interventions in relation to advances in science and technology, for example gene therapies, vaccinations, equipment or medical devices that can enhance or even prolong life. There are different types of innovation, and they do not always need to be 'big ideas':

- Product – changes in products or services.
- Process – changes in the ways products or solutions are created and delivered.
- Position – changes in the context in which products or solutions are introduced.
- Paradigm – changes in the way that we think about things.

Innovation has to be more than a simple improvement in performance – it needs to be radical in the way it sets about tackling a problem or be a real advancement in the way that we think or do something. Conversely, there is an important role for what is termed 'reverse innovation' – this is the decommissioning of an activity that is shown to have no added value or that has been replaced by something new or better.

> Visit the Health Foundation website (https://www.health.org.uk/funding-and-partnerships/funding-programmes/funding-for-improvement-projects), which showcases funding opportunities and actual service improvement and evidence-based innovation projects led by a range of NHS and provider organisations.
>
> Look at the sort of things that are highlighted as being innovative practice. A lot of the innovations are centred on the use of information technology and advances in treatments and medicines. Think about your own practice. What do you consider to be innovative? It may be something as simple as a new way of working.

Activity 10.3

Furthermore, innovation involves horizon scanning by looking to the future in relation to emerging issues or diseases, such as the recognition and alert around COVID-19 prior to the global pandemic. Changes in healthcare delivery and improvement in methodology, sharing of good practice and ensuring expertise and advice are disseminated support innovation in the way care could be improved by using new approaches and technologies. In addition, there could be engagement with institutions and nations where innovation and research might involve collaboration across a range of disciplines or populations to advance practice (Royal College of General Practitioners, 2021).

Innovation is also represented in the way Integrated Care Systems (NHS England, 2021) have been developed, with place-based hubs meaning care is closer to home, more accessible, reducing costs in terms of greater access to treatment and reduced 'Did not attend' rates, with enhanced patient outcomes and experience. In turn, this seeks to coordinate services and improve population health, reducing inequalities with a range of services and partners across private voluntary and statutory agencies able to provide integrated care for patients and communities (NHS Improvement, 2021).

Another feature or benefit of Integrated Care Systems is the minimalisation of referral processes, with greater communication and knowledge around services and accessibility, inhibiting the referral to services that is bounced back for using the wrong form, referring to the wrong service, with the wrong referral criteria for example, leading to, at best, delayed assessment and intervention, to, at worst, risk of deterioration and loss of the patient to the system with risk to safety. Integrated care systems priorities, drawn from the

NHS Long Term Plan, include integration of primary and community services to facilitate joined-up services between multidisciplinary teams, a proactive role in population health and prevention, services drawing on local resources through community, voluntary and independent sectors, to include public services, with multi-specialty interventions across care disciplines, for example, mental health and physical health, health and social care, across the lifespan (Health Education England, 2021).

Leadership goes hand in hand with innovation and this should focus on systems leadership, enabling trusting relationships, collaboration between organisational and professional boundaries and shared system goals. Compassionate, inclusive leadership involves paying attention to those you lead, understanding issues presented to them and taking action to help (NHS Leadership Academy, 2016). Effective, inclusive leadership behaviours initiate just learning cultures, engaging staff, patients and carers in generating service improvement as well as valuing diversity and challenging power imbalances (King's Fund, 2016). Research shows that such cultures are sustained by organisations that have:

- an unwavering commitment to providing safe, high-quality care;
- a commitment to effective, efficient, high-quality performance;
- behaviours characterised by support, compassion and inclusion for all patients and staff;
- ways of working that focus on continuous learning, quality improvement and innovation;
- enthusiastic cooperation, teamworking and support within and across boundaries.

(West et al., 2014)

Patient outcomes and experience (Mohanna, 2017; NHS Constitution, 2021; NMC, 2018b) remain the focus of all service transformation initiatives. Even where cost reduction and service reconfiguration impact on delivery, the focus should be equity of access, reducing unwarranted variation, ensuring efficiency, health and wellbeing, care and quality while also focusing on funding and efficiency. Regular scrutiny of effectiveness is critical to improvement and innovation over timescales to monitor but also modify aims and measurement of success to avoid risk of the project failing.

Patients, service users and communities should be involved as equal partners in redesigning and improving processes and systems. In this sense, EBP is evolving as evidence is also acquired from patient engagement and involvement, what works best for the public and demand on services as well as evidence-based interventions and new approaches to care delivery, including consultation through technology, reducing risk and cost to the public in the way they access care. A collaborative approach can improve communication, save time, reduce duplication of effort, improve working relationships and provide a better experience for people who use health and social care services (NHS England & NHS Improvement, 2019).

GETTING EVIDENCE INTO PRACTICE

EBP is an essential element to moving practice forward and an important component in service development, innovation and improvement. While EBP is generally accepted as something to aspire to, in reality changes to practices are not easily made. Understanding the complexities of change and, in particular, achieving sustainable change is useful when thinking about getting evidence into practice. Timmins et al. (2012) found that a number of issues impacted on nurses' use of research findings in practice. These relate to a lack of time to engage in EBP activities such as finding relevant up-to-date research; limited skills in relation to application of research to practice; and a perceived lack of support from colleagues and managers coupled with an apparent reluctance to adopt new practices by some. The time between evidence being generated and practice being adopted in a setting could be significant. Often practices will be considered safe, having been based on evidence, but frequently this will be out-of-date theory.

Getting evidence into practice is not a straightforward activity. The reasons why valid evidence and clinical guidelines are not routinely adopted into practice are often complex and involve both the individual and organisation. Nibbelink and Brewer (2018) suggest that nurses prefer to rely on experiential sources of knowledge. This type of knowledge is valued because it is specific to the context in which nurses work, as well as readily accessible and patient centred. Research, on the other hand, tends to be seen as less easy to access, and often not specifically relevant to the sorts of issues nurses are faced with. Nurses also appear to prefer others (such as nurse specialists) to provide them with research evidence rather than seek it out themselves.

In the late 1990s, the King's Fund (2000) was asked to look at the effectiveness of different approaches to putting evidence into practice. They looked at 17 London-based projects that sought to implement evidence-based change and identified four key factors for putting evidence into practice. They found that:

- resources need to be sufficient;
- the proposed change needs to offer benefits of real interest to staff who have to change;
- enough of the right people need to be on board early enough; and
- the approach needs to be interactive and relate research to current practice.

Barkham and Mellor-Clark (2003) argued that the most difficult part of making a change is getting people to let go of their usual practices. Often there is what MacGuire (1990) has described as the 'shifting sands syndrome': at each point of the process of change, barriers are identified by participants to prevent anyone taking the next step ('It can't be done because…'). People prefer what is 'familiar' to them and are therefore often resistant to what they see as a threat to their normal activities and likely to increase their levels of stress. McPhail (1997) refers to this as 'comfort zones' which nurses have developed over time and are reluctant to change unless they become disenchanted with particular established practices. Moving people out of their comfort zone is not an easy task and can be at the heart of whether change is successful or not. Concerns may relate to beliefs (either real or imagined) about what the change will mean for them and where it will come from.

The advent of EBP has brought with it the term 'implementing evidence-based practices', which considers how evidence – and in particular research – can be applied in the practice setting. 'Knowledge translation', 'knowledge/evidence utilisation' and 'research implementation' are also used to describe the processes involved in applying knowledge/evidence to a practice setting. Just as there is a plethora of terms there is also a range of approaches through which it can sometimes appear difficult to navigate. However, the central premise for all of these terms and models is the need to ensure that health professionals' clinical practice is effective and based on sound and current evidence. Much has been written about **change management**, where various theoretical models outlining the process and mechanisms that can be used for making changes to behaviours and practices are described. Changing care delivery and individuals' behaviours and approaches takes time and effort. It is important to be thoroughly prepared before trying to instigate changes. There is no single best way of introducing new evidence into practice, as the type of change required will often dictate the approach to be used.

Activity 10.4

Imagine that you have been told you need to change a particular aspect of your practice. What feelings would this evoke and what would be your most likely response?

Conversely, what factors would make you think of changing your practice?

Often change is brought about by personal endeavour and aligned to personal goals. People have different interests, motivators and tolerance – which influences behaviour and how people respond to change. Evidence suggests that health and social care staff are motivated to change by (King's Fund, 2015):

- savings in time;
- savings in money;
- improved patient care;
- professional development (and this has been found to be particularly valued by nurses);
- changes that address their operational concerns (particularly in their own priority areas);
- and changes that show benefit for all of the group (so those all round win/win situations – the 'why wouldn't you?').

When thinking about change it's often worth checking out how this affects you personally (see Appendix 8 Personal Development Plan). Does the proposed change sit with your goals, drives and ambitions?

In making a change at the individual level there is still a need to consider patient preferences, identifying whether (NHS, 2019):

- the change is appropriate to the patients' expressed preferences;
- patients are aware of their options in terms of care delivery and able to make an informed choice;
- it is ethically and culturally acceptable to the patient;
- it is practicable in the context you practise in;
- you have the knowledge, skills and resources to implement the change.

There is also a need to discuss changes with practice colleagues to ensure that actions do not cause friction or difficulties within the care team and do not run counter to the care philosophy of practice (Fulford et al., 2012).

In order to facilitate change, there needs to be an understanding as to the complexities of health and social care and recognition that neither is static but evolving. Central to this whole process is the patient. It is, therefore, important that any intervention or improvement should be based on the needs of those that use the service. There is a need to work flexibly and across different groups and to look at the reasons that have tended to underline poor practice, these being:

- inconsistent standards – between practitioners, departments and organisations;
- barriers between services;
- inflexible, unresponsive services;
- over-centralisation and the disempowerment of patients and staff.

(Page and Hammer, 2002)

When thinking about change we are encouraged to focus on the three areas below:

- Structures refer to the geography and lay out of facilities and equipment, organisational boundaries, roles and responsibilities, teams, committees and working groups, targets and goals.
- Processes refer to patient journeys, care pathways, educational processes, funding flows, recruitment of staff, procurement and supporting processes such as ordering, delivery and dispensing.
- Patterns refer to patterns of thinking and behaviours, conversations, relationships, communication and learning, decision making, conflict and power.

(NHS Institute for Innovation and Improvement, 2005)

Before any change can be initiated a plan is required that identifies the reason why the change is needed and how it will be carried out. There are a number of improvement frameworks and models to guide the clinician in practice. All make use of data to evaluate needs and opportunities, refine solutions and monitor outcomes. A popular model is the Model of Effective Implementation. This follows a straightforward and systematic process whereby information and data are collected in support of the proposed change, the change is planned for and then introduced, following which it is evaluated. Grol et al. (2013) offered the following model for effective implementation:

1. Research findings/guidelines (the evidence is gathered).
2. Matching problems identified or best practices (current practice is evaluated against 'best practice').
3. Describing specific change targets.
4. Analysis of target group, current practice and context.
5. Development/selection of strategies (a plan is put in place).
6. Development and execution of implementation plan.
7. Continuous evaluation and adapting plan.

It is clear that any attempt to change should be planned for and actively managed. Any proposed change needs to involve all those who will be affected by it, and this, in turn, will inform the circumstances in which the evidence is disseminated and introduced into the practice setting. Dissemination activities by themselves are unlikely to lead to changes in behaviour; however, this should not be taken to mean that raising awareness of the messages underpinning proposed changes is unimportant. Implementation has its own specific areas for consideration. Metz et al. (2007) suggest that there are three types of implementation:

1. Paper – where policies are in place but no changes to practice actually occur.
2. Fragmented – new structures are put in place but not targeted at the right people; therefore, those involved are unable to develop the necessary skills and again practice remains unchanged.
3. Impact implementation – where strategies and structures are appropriate and are designed specifically to ensure practice change.

In implementing change there is a need to ensure that all these have been taken into consideration and addressed before attempting to make a change. There is also a need to check progress frequently and ensure feedback is given to people at regular intervals, so they are aware of progress and any issues that have arisen. If changes to practice are to be sustained and the practices implemented remain in place, there is a further need to ensure that the necessary resources are maintained, and people are rewarded for doing a good job.

The PARiHS (Promoting Action on Research Implementation in Health Services) framework developed by an RCN project group (Rycroft-Malone, 2004) draws together three elements that are thought to be central to the success of making changes to practice:

1. Evidence – its clarity.
2. Context – its quality.
3. Facilitation – type needed.

Activity 10.5

Visit the National Collaborating Centre for Methods and Tools, McMaster University, Canada and review the PARiHS framework for implementing research into practice using the following link: www.nccmt.ca/knowledge-repositories/search/85. Review how research has been introduced into your clinical environment using the framework. To what extent did the research impact on clinical practice? Would you say that its implementation had been a success? What did success look like?

For change to be successfully brought about, the evidence on which changes are to be based needs to be high quality, valued and viewed as relevant by both the clinical staff and patients/service users. Grol and Grimshaw (2003) noted the characteristics of the evidence can have a major influence on whether it is integrated into practice, and that some forms of evidence are easier to integrate into practice than others. If evidence reflects widespread concerns in relation to particular practices, or is seen as supporting professional group values, then it is more likely to be adopted. The quality of evidence also impacts on uptake, for example guidelines that are clear, explicit and straightforward are more likely to be implemented.

Once a body of evidence on a particular issue which has implications for practice has been identified, there is a need to evaluate and synthesise this evidence to identify what needs to be done in relation to the specific area of interest (Fineout-Overholt et al., 2010). Once the relevant evidence has been critically appraised and a summary sheet of the relevant papers created (see Appendix 9) this will give an indication of the key aspects of the evidence and which papers are or are not applicable to practice. The implications of integrating these findings into practice and whether or not this has broader implications for others will need to be considered. Any proposed changes will require careful planning and should be discussed with colleagues to ensure the identification of any potential difficulties with the process of implementation.

The context in which care is delivered is itself constantly changing. Patients come and go, their conditions change or may deteriorate rapidly, and working with other healthcare professionals brings its own complexities. If change is to be made against this sort of background there is a need for individuals to feel valued, for necessary resources to be readily available and for effective teamwork practices to be in place.

In implementing change there is a need to ensure that all these factors have been taken into consideration and addressed before attempting to make a change. There is also a need to check progress frequently and ensure feedback is given to people at regular intervals so they are aware of progress and any issues that have arisen. If changes to practice are to be sustained and the practices implemented to remain in place, there is a further need to ensure that the necessary resources are maintained, and people are rewarded for doing a good job.

The Process of Implementing Evidence-based Practices

Identifying potential barriers to getting evidence into practice is an important first step when thinking about introducing change. Rycroft-Malone et al. (2004) identified four main reasons for the under-use of research in practice: (1) the clinician's inability to interpret research findings; (2) lack of organisational support; (3) research seen as lacking clinical credibility; (4) clinicians preferring a specialist to tell them of the latest developments. These factors were similar to those found by Alatawi et al. (2020), that: (1) lack of support and supervision; (2) lack of training and education; (3) limited resources; and (4) time restrictions were the biggest obstacles to getting evidence into practice.

There are various models available to guide the process of changing practice (see Table 10.1 for examples). They all have certain aspects in common, including the need for planning, implementation and evaluation strategies to be in place.

An approach commonly used with NHS service improvement initiatives is the PDSA cycle (Plan, Do, Study, Act). This is based on the work of Deming (1986) and reflects the scientific process of hypothesis (Plan), experiment (Do) and evaluate (Study). See Table 10.2 for an overview of this. You might also consider that this is also like a nursing approach to patient care: hypothesis (plan) [assess need], experiment (do) [implement care], evaluate (study) [reassess/evaluate care], act [continue to implement care which delivers positive outcomes for the individual].

Table 10.1 Models for promoting change

Brady and Lewin (2007)	Lewin (1951)	Metz et al. (2007)
1. **Plan** – involve all affected by the change Identify outcomes Pilot proposals Identify motivators 2. **Implement** – establish a realistic time line with built-in evaluation points 3. **Correct** – be flexible and address issues as they arise 4. **Communicate** – use multiple ways of keeping people informed 5. **Evaluate** – identify impact of changes for both professionals and service users	1. **Unfreeze** – recognition of need for change 2. **Moving** – making the change by altering behaviours or activities 3. **Refreeze** – embedding the changes in practice	1. **Exploration** – change/implementation ideas considered 2. **Preparation** – resources needed identified and made available 3. **Early implementation** – initial adjustments to implement practices made 4. **Full implementation** – all staff have appropriate level of competency and change is fully embedded in activities 5. **Sustainability** – skills, knowledge and resources are maintained at required level to ensure changes remain in place 6. **Innovation** – consideration of adaptations and other changes required

Table 10.2 PDSA cycle

	Stage
Plan	What are the objectives?
	Who will do what, when, where and how?
	How will you evaluate progress/what data will you collect?
Do	Implement plan
	Note any problems/issues that arise throughout the implementation
Study	Analyse data collected
	Compare data with objectives
	Identify what you have learnt
Act	What do you want to achieve next?
	How will you do this?

Iles and Sutherland (2001) suggest that it is important that these aspects are not seen as being separate and discrete stages that are undertaken in isolation. It is likely, no matter how thorough the planning, that issues will arise which have not been considered; therefore, planning must remain a continuous process. The implementation phase needs to be evaluated at all points to ensure that what is intended to happen, does indeed do so.

As issues arise, further planning and then implementation will be needed, with an evaluation of the impact of adjustments made. As Schön (1994) describes, there are areas of professional practice where evidence can be easily used to support practice – the high hard ground; however, more frequently practice occurs in 'messy' and 'swampy lowlands' where there are challenging problems which will frequently impact on the rigorous application of evidence to practice.

The planning stage usually involves what is known as a diagnostic analysis. As Nickols (2016) suggests, change is a problem-solving activity, which usually starts with a diagnosis of the problem, allowing goals to be identified and strategies by which these can be achieved put in place. The 'problem' considered in relation to EBP is the moving from one practice to another and, therefore, the diagnostic analysis will involve a consideration of the area or context within which change is to be made. The idea is to identify any barriers and organisational and/or professional issues which must be taken into account before any attempt is made to implement change. This also allows for the identification of the gap between what is currently happening and what the vision for the future is. Highlighting the gap makes planning the implementation easier and also reduces the likelihood of unforeseen problems and barriers to changing practices arising.

One of the simplest and easiest approaches to consider the issues around making a change is to use a SWOT analysis – Strengths, Weaknesses, Opportunities and Threats. An alternative to SWOT is the 7S model presented in Table 10.3.

Table 10.3 7S model

Element	Features
Staff	What is needed – number, skill mix, characteristics (attitudes, values, etc.)?
Skills	What is needed and what are available in relation to: • clinical/technical skills? • interpersonal skills? • managerial skills? • research/EBP skills?
Structure	What are the current features of the organisation? What is needed? What is the 'fit' between the two?
Systems	What is in place and what is needed?
Strategy	What is the plan? What are the priorities?
Style (management)	What is the current style? Does this fit with what is needed to achieve the planned changes?
Shared beliefs	What beliefs and values are present? What is needed to achieve the planned change? Is there a gap between the two?

Activity 10.6

Identify an area of practice that you would like to change and use either a SWOT (a template is provided in Appendix 10) or the 7S model to identify the issues you would need to consider.

An alternative to these two models is the 'how, what and why' approach. These question types reflect the various approaches to change that different people take within organisations – namely their 'mindset'. Working through these questions can help to address all the issues that need to be considered and planned for.

- How do I get colleagues to change from X to Y intervention?
- What do I want to achieve, what changes have to be made, what will indicate success?
- Why is X intervention used and why do we need to change to Y?

Activity 10.7

Consider the SWOT or 7S analysis you undertook in relation to your chosen area of practice. Does the 'how, what, why' approach provide information you hadn't considered?

Once all the issues that may impact on implementing change and the resources needed have been identified, planning how to make the change is undertaken. There is a need here to set realistic goals, to identify a timeline and draw up an implementation strategy. Changing practices takes time, and all those that the change will affect should be involved, with time to ensure there is adequate consultation and planning.

McLean (2011) contends there is also a need to manage the psychological impact of making the transition from one practice to another. As transitions involve 'endings' it is necessary to consider how best to manage these. She suggested a five-step model, which acknowledges the psychological impact implicit in moving from one practice to another. Often, people experience anxiety and worry about the implications of changes, and without a clear vision of why practices are 'ending' may view previous ways of working through 'rose tinted glasses'. There are three phases to transition: 'ending', when 'old' practices are stopping; neutral, where 'old' practices have not completely finished and 'new' practices are not fully embedded; and a 'beginning' phase when the new practice is fully implemented. McLean (2011) asserted that a transition facilitator and/or team should be set up to ensure the transition runs smoothly.

Once the change has been fully integrated into practice there is a need to formally evaluate the implementation of the practice, identifying whether the change has had an appropriate impact on care, the lessons learnt and whether further innovations are needed. It is crucial to know whether or not the intended point has actually been arrived at and whether the planned change is an improvement on previous practices. Evaluation needs to be planned as part of the process of introducing new practices and taking decisions in the planning phase as to what is intended to be evaluated – the effectiveness of the practice, the processes used, the impact of the changes, or all three.

Practice development and improvement uses research and theory in a way that is sensitive to practice issues on the ground. Practice development methodologies address:

- facilitated approaches to improving practice;
- development of leadership attributes and skills;
- development of team effectiveness and new ways of working;
- evaluation of changes in workplace culture and the context of practice delivery.

Methodologies include, for example, action research, evaluation research, investigative enquiry, practice enquiry, integrative enquiry and evidence-based practice.

It is clear that any attempt to change should be based on evidence, use a systematic approach and involve planning, active monitoring and evaluation. Any proposed change – for example, a change of practice based on new research – would involve the development of an appropriate dissemination and implementation strategy, clearly articulating the need for change and the strength of evidence on which it is based. This should include plans to monitor and evaluate the degree to which the proposed change has been achieved and its effects, together with methods to maintain and reinforce any change, including the removal of barriers to change. Greater insight is needed into the personal skills and attributes of those being asked to make the change as well as those being asked to lead the change. It may be useful to consider sharing the experience of making changes with a wider audience, writing up the project for publication or presenting it at a conference. A wider dissemination through publication/conference presentation may help others struggling with similar problems, while at the same time adding to the evidence base for nursing practice.

Activity 10.8

The National Institute for Health and Care Excellence has produced a document on the principles for putting evidence-based guidance into practice, which you can access using the following link: www.nice.org.uk/Media/Default/About/what-we-do/Into-practice/Principles-for-putting-evidence-based-guidance-into-practice.pdf

Read through the guidance, which covers much of what we have discussed in the chapter. Make sure to click on the practical step links in the document as they then take you off to additional resources. Well worth a visit.

Summary

- In order to move practice forward there needs to be a commitment to innovation and improvement and the development of practice.
- Service development helps to identify best practice by focusing on continuous improvement.

(Continued)

- Both innovation and improvement imply doing; change is an active process.
- The transferring of evidence into practice is a complex activity, which takes time and effort.
- Comfort zones develop over time and change is unlikely unless nurses are motivated to change established practices.
- A shared vision is needed if change is to be successful and people need to have the skills and to see the benefits of implementing a new practice.
- Change can occur on a personal, team, organisation, national or even global level.
- Strategies and structures need to be designed specifically to ensure practice changes are sustained.

FURTHER READING

Backhouse, A. and Ogunlayi, F. (2020) 'Quality improvement into practice', *The British Medical Journal, 368*: m865. doi:10.1136/bmj.m865
NHS England (2017) *Building a Knowledge Enabled NHS for the Future*. London: NHS England.
The Health Foundation (2021) *Quality Improvement Made Simple: What Everyone Should Know about Health Care Quality Improvement*. London: The Health Foundation.

USEFUL WEBLINKS

The Health Foundation: this organisation has a specific interest in the implementation of evidence into health and social care practice. Take time to explore their site: www.health.org.uk

The Point of Care Foundation: this charitable organisation works to provide the tools and support for individuals and organisations to bring about change in clinical practice. www.pointofcarefoundation.org.uk

11

Clinical Academic Careers

Ros Kane and Christine Jackson

Learning Outcomes

By the end of the chapter, you will be able to:

- briefly describe the historical context around the move to degree-level education in nursing, midwifery and allied health;
- define what is meant by the term clinical academic;
- identify potential routes to becoming a clinical academic;
- discuss the contribution that clinical academic staff can make to evidence-based practice.

INTRODUCTION

The engagement of healthcare staff in research has been shown to be associated with improved healthcare performance (Boaz et al., 2015). Indeed, the ability of healthcare professionals to engage in critical enquiry and implement research findings is imperative for the application of evidence to practice, and there are many examples of where this makes a significant difference to care experience and clinical effectiveness (Health Education England [HEE], 2015). Historically, the phrase 'theory–practice gap' has frequently been used in healthcare literature and has been referred to as 'the inability to relate and implement ideological knowledge gained in education to the realities of modern-day healthcare practice' (Clark and Holmes, 2007). This has been shown to apply both to students, when transferring the skills taught in the academic setting to clinical practice, and to newly qualified staff, transitioning into the role (Monaghan, 2015), and also to more experienced qualified staff amongst whom, it is argued, there may also be a lack of proficiency in both their clinical skills and critical thinking abilities (Greenway et al., 2019). Despite the considerable history of theory development in healthcare, nursing in particular has consistently struggled to reconcile theoretical reality and practice realities (Zieber and Wojtowicz, 2019). Acknowledging that the term 'theory–practice gap' is often without consistent definition, Greenway et al. (2019) have contributed to our understanding of this concept and redefined it in specific reference to nursing as: '*The gap between the theoretical knowledge and the practical application of nursing, most often expressed as a negative entity, with adverse consequences.*' Research and evidence-based practice underpin the delivery of high-quality patient care in the clinical setting so arguably the continuing development of clinical academic careers, including from the outset of undergraduate education (research placements for students are now widely advocated for example), is one strategy towards bridging this 'gap' and equipping healthcare professionals with the skills needed to begin to generate, interpret and implement evidence into clinical practice. However, developing the research capacity and capability of nurses, midwives and allied health professionals requires a commitment from across sectors and through the managerial hierarchy within organisations: embedding clinical academic careers within a healthcare organisation is challenging (Gerrish and Chapman, 2017). Examples are emerging of successful development of the necessary support infrastructure needed to encourage and develop healthcare professionals to follow a clinical academic career pathway, including clinical academic partnerships between universities and healthcare institutions (Stricktland, 2017).

The drive to establish clinical academic careers in the United Kingdom has gained momentum in recent years, facilitated to a great extent by opportunities and funding offered by the Higher Education England/National Institute for Health Research integrated clinical academic pathway, which now provides an increasingly successful way of bridging the theory–practice gap as well as supporting the nursing, midwifery and allied healthcare workforce in the delivery of evidence- and values-based practice. Clinical academics maintain their practice role while also carrying out research, placing them in a unique position to make connections between research and clinical practice, and to pose new research questions arising from their clinical observations and experience. Professionals who develop a clinical academic career can play a significant role in cultural and behavioural change within organisations and are hallmarked by their leadership potential around the area of evidence-based practice. Training paths for clinical academic roles have existed across the UK since 2006 and clinical research is a fast-growing career pathway for many healthcare workers. However, relative to medicine, the role is still in its infancy. Aspiring clinical academics, despite many recent developments, still face a range of challenges in balancing the clinical and research aspects of their careers, and in applying for and succeeding in opportunities afforded to them. A new report published by the Council of Deans of Health identifies significant barriers as well as opportunities for developing more nurses, midwives and allied health professionals working in both clinical practice and academic research in the UK, citing in particular a lack of clear career entry points for early career researchers, the lack of a clear model of career progression and insufficient post-doctoral posts (Baltruks and Callaghan, 2018). The report goes on to call for the creation of robust frameworks for clinical academic research career pathways in all four nations, support for clinical academics through mentoring schemes, strong programmes for continuing professional development and dedicated PhD and post-doctoral training programmes (Baltruks and Callaghan, 2018).

Many clinical academic staff must still carve out their own career pathways and influence their workplaces to enable and support their dual practice/research role, so developing as autonomous practitioners. Influencing and leadership skills are key, as well as developing excellent research skills applied to the particular contexts in which they are working.

As with the expansion of the nurse's role (see Chapter 1), the introduction of evidence-based practice challenged the way in which clinicians are educated and supported. In 2006, a key document from the Department of Health in England set priority areas for modernisation, which included updating career pathways and choices (DH, 2006). This modernisation programme recognised that healthcare was changing and so too was the healthcare workforce. By the mid-2000s, nursing had become an all-degree profession across the UK. One of the key outcomes from the transition to degree-level qualification was the need to refocus academic research and clinical practice through the creation of opportunities for an innovative career pathway that combined a strong clinical focus together with the benefits of research training. Evidence-based practice was promoted as a means of facilitating this change and fed directly into the development of specialist practitioner roles; for example, non-medical prescribing, practice education and teaching. The role of the clinical academic can be seen as a further development in response to these changes in practice and education. With the generation, interpretation and implementation of evidence being key concerns, clinical academics are well placed to contribute to the improvement of practice; but in order for nurses and other health professionals to engage in research activity, they need to have access to appropriate education and training. Lifelong learning and continuing professional development are important concepts and have a central part in developing a competent and flexible workforce. Nurses and other healthcare professionals need to be made aware of the real opportunities contained within the clinical academic role and how to access them.

This chapter examines the historical development of the clinical academic role and outlines examples of current practice. Presented below is a description of the historical context and subsequent policies leading to the development of the current clinical academic career pathways in England for nurses, midwives and allied health professionals. Allied health professions refer to those professions located within the statutory framework of the Health and Care Professions Council (HCPC). There are currently (2021) 15 health and care professions sitting within the HCPC (see: www.hcpc-uk.co.uk/about-us/who-we-regulate/ for a full list and additional information about the role of each profession).

WHO ARE CLINICAL ACADEMICS?

It is important to define what is meant by a clinical academic within nursing, midwifery and allied healthcare professions. The definition used here was formulated by the National Institute for Health Research (NIHR) and adopted by the Association of UK University Hospitals (AUKUH) for use with their online resource, *Transforming Healthcare* (2016), which provides a focal point and guide when thinking about the implementation and development of clinical academics, and is as follows:

> Clinical academics are clinically active health researchers. They work in health and social care as clinicians to improve, maintain, or recover health while in parallel researching new ways of delivering better outcomes for the patients they treat and care for. Clinical academics also work in higher education institutions (HEIs) while providing clinical expertise to health and social care. Because they remain clinically active, their research is grounded in the day to day issues of their patients and service. This dual role also allows the clinical academic to combine their clinical and research career rather than having to choose between the two. (Association of UK University Hospitals (AUKUH), 2016: 9)

Activity 11.1

Before reading any further, take time out to identify a clinical academic who might be working in your area. 'Interview' them and reflect on their role; is it a career that might interest you?

The case study below details the experience of a senior academic who previously worked clinically as a therapeutic radiographer. The experience is very typical of clinicians with an interest in developing their research skills, prior to the introduction of the concept of a clinical academic career and the availability of training opportunities.

Case study 11.1

'I always enjoyed my clinical work and the rapport one develops with patients. The drive you have, to help and support patients through a rewarding career in healthcare, never leaves you but at the same time I wanted something more. That is why I moved from clinical practice into academia. For a number of years, I enjoyed the very different challenges that academia brought and almost 30 years after qualifying, I gained my PhD. Looking back on what I, my colleagues, and peers considered a successful career, my one regret was that I lost my clinical focus and my clinical skills. I missed the patients too. If I were qualifying today, I would hope to take a different career pathway. I would have applied for a clinical academic position and would have undertaken a clinically based PhD study much earlier in my career. This would have allowed me to retain a clinical focus with patients and in addition act as a role model for future aspiring clinical academics. Perhaps, I would go on to either lead a research group or become a consultant practitioner.'

Senior academic, therapeutic radiographer

HISTORICAL PERSPECTIVES ON THE DEVELOPMENT OF EDUCATION AND TRAINING FOR NURSES, MIDWIVES AND ALLIED HEALTH PROFESSIONALS

Nursing as a profession has been recognised for over 150 years, with the first training school established in 1860, the Nightingale Training School for Nurses at St Thomas' Hospital in London. One of the first institutions to teach nursing and midwifery as formal professions, it was dedicated to communicating the philosophy and practice of its founder and patron, Florence Nightingale. Nursing qualifications later moved from certificated to diploma training and the majority of training schools were under the control of Health Authorities (the then government agency that was responsible for NHS care in a particular area), with the academic staff in the schools of nursing remaining as NHS employees. A similar approach was taken by those professions considered under the umbrella of allied health, including radiographers, physiotherapists and occupational therapists. Training schools for allied health professions were becoming established throughout the latter part of the twentieth century and were largely single discipline, geographically attached to the larger hospitals, with academic staff drawn from clinical practice who, as with nursing and midwifery, remained as NHS employees (though notable exceptions were the Universities of Edinburgh and Salford where degree programmes in radiography were offered as early as the 1960s).

This structure afforded very clear and direct opportunities for the clinical departments, clinical staff and training schools to work effectively as a unit supporting the students. This close working partnership ensured the availability of opportunities for staff in the training schools to retain their clinical skills and knowledge. Clinical and training heads of service were mutually supportive and often served on hospital management committees together. This encouraged a two-way flow of expertise and information, which in turn benefited the students. However, students – particularly in nursing and midwifery – were considered part of the workforce rather than being supernumerary and this was beginning to cause concern for the professional and registration bodies in place at this time.

Criticisms of the NHS training school structure began to emerge in the 1980s and were wide-ranging. Concerns were expressed by the then Department of Health and Social Services and professional bodies that undertaking diploma-level qualifications through a single-discipline training programme was becoming an outdated approach to training students across healthcare. Considerable discussion took place about the lack of research utilisation in clinical practice and the need to change traditional working practices in keeping with contemporary thinking and a changing health and economic landscape.

The majority of training schools had no links with higher education institutions and were not in a position to benefit from wider academic expertise or multidisciplinary education at Bachelor level through to Master's and PhD qualifications. During the 1980s, staff in training schools, where the majority held diploma-level and higher professional qualifications, began seeking additional academic qualifications via university programmes. This exposure to the higher education system and the graduate community was providing, for many training staff, an insight into and experience of a wider, formalised academic environment where the principles of learning centred on education rather than training.

In nursing, students were not supernumerary to the clinical nursing workforce, which meant they were often considered as an unqualified member of staff and learnt much of their practice from direct clinical experience. The move to higher education and to degree-level nurse education was arguably an attempt to develop a culture of research awareness, and to provide support and guidance in the development of research skills and the application of research in clinical practice. It also allowed nursing to be placed on a similar footing to other professions (such as physiotherapy), which had embraced degree-based education much earlier. Similar moves are being seen today with paramedic and operating department practitioner training now also being taught at degree-level.

MOVING TOWARDS GRADUATE PROFESSIONS: POLICY INITIATIVES (1980–2000)

Nursing and midwifery

In the 1980s and 1990s, pre-registration courses were criticised for their failure to adequately equip students with the necessary knowledge and skills to assume the role of a qualified nurse (Bradshaw and Merriman, 2008; Glen, 2009; Maben and Macleod-Clark, 1998). This provided impetus for the radical reorganisation of nurse education in the UK and the introduction of a new nursing curriculum (Jasper, 1996). The two decades between 1980 to 2000 saw a defined shift in focus for education and training programmes in nursing and midwifery. In 1986, the United Kingdom Central Council for Nursing, Midwifery and Health Visiting (UKCC) (the then professional governing body in the UK), launched Project 2000, which aimed to move nursing education into the higher education sector and create a single tier of Registered General Nurses (RGN) in contrast to the previous two-tier registration: the State Enrolled Nurse (SEN), which required a two-year training programme, and the State Registered Nurse (SRN), which a required a three-year diploma programme of study. It proposed to educate a 'knowledgeable doer' capable of both giving and supervising nursing care. The aim was to produce a mature and confident practitioner who was able to accept responsibility, think analytically and flexibly, be able to recognise a need for further preparation, and was willing to engage in self-development (UKCC, 1986). Project 2000 became the driver for the transfer of schools of nursing and midwifery into higher education institutes and set a route to enable the diploma qualification to be phased out and replaced by pre-registration undergraduate programmes in nursing and midwifery. Nurse training, therefore, moved away from the traditional 'apprentice-style' education to a diploma-level curriculum built upon firm theoretical knowledge (Glen, 2009).

In the late 1990s, Project 2000 came under scrutiny as experienced health professionals expressed concerns about levels of fitness to practise among newly qualified nurses (Gerrish, 2000; Higgins et al., 2010; Maben and Macleod-Clark, 1998). These concerns led to an examination of the Project 2000 curriculum and the formation of two documents, namely *Making a Difference* (DH, 1999) (which also applied to midwifery education) and *Fitness for Practice* (UKCC, 1999), and also the publication of recommendations to strengthen pre- and post-registration education and training in the UK (Higgins et al., 2010). *Making a Difference* (DH, 1999) and *Fitness for Practice* (UKCC, 1999) provided the foundation for new curricula and the move towards all-degree education (Higgins et al., 2010).

Allied health professions

Although there were some early successes in terms of developing pre-registration degree programmes (the first undergraduate programme in physiotherapy was validated at the University of Ulster in 1976), the majority of the other allied health professions had to wait considerably longer (Price, 2009).

During the late 1970s, the Boards of the Council for Professions Supplementary to Medicine (CPSM), now known as the Health and Care Professions Council (HCPC), together with representatives across education and health from the four UK countries, set up the Higher and Further Education Working Party to consider pertinent issues in healthcare education and training. In 1979, the working party published *The Next Decade* (1979), which made 60 recommendations. One of these was the transfer of funding from the health sector to education, which would bring allied health professions in line with the funding mechanisms in medicine and dentistry. This report might be considered as the impetus for the professional bodies to begin reviewing existing pre-registration qualifications with a view to moving towards a graduate entry for allied health professions. However, it took several more years of debate and discussions with stakeholders across health and education before the professions began to see progress towards approvals for undergraduate pre-registration programmes.

The publication of *Working for Patients* (DH, 1989), on the future of education and training, outlined the case for radical reforms of the organisation of NHS training schools with a view to transferring the management and funding mechanisms to the education sector. This working paper provided the impetus for all allied health professions in existence at this time, along with their professional bodies and the CPSM, to work with the then national degree awarding body, the Council for National Academic Awards (CNAA), to validate and accredit pre-registration undergraduate programmes.

> Take time out to search the history of your profession and how it has developed. What is expected from the professional of the future? How much expectation is there that research should be integral to clinical activity? How much preparation and assistance are offered to support the development of research skills and expertise?
>
> **Activity 11.2**

DEVELOPING RESEARCH SKILLS

History and policy context for clinical academic careers

The previous section provided a brief overview of the reforms to pre-registration education and training programmes for nurses, midwives and allied health professionals, detailing the move from the health sector into the higher education system in the UK. Education within the university environment brings recognised benefits. Undergraduate students are now exposed to a multidisciplinary environment and are part of a wider cohort of the university student body with a national voice. The students have access to world-class educational technology to support their learning and are within a research-rich environment.

Healthcare academics within schools of nursing, midwifery and allied health are drawn largely from the professions. Healthcare education must retain a strong professional focus and be able to measure professional competence, and students must be confirmed as fit to practise at qualification. The students benefit from research-informed teaching and are afforded opportunities to engage in research prior to qualification.

Moving to an all-degree profession was arguably one of the key actions in modernising nursing. It not only raised the standing of the profession but the expectations of its workforce, including the ability to engage in and implement the findings of research, and this has been reflected in a number of national reports. Recent reviews of educational provision have re-ignited the debate about the content of programmes, with specific reference to the coverage of research topics. For example, in England, The Shape of Caring review (2012), commissioned by Health Education England in partnership with the Nursing and Midwifery Council, published recommendations for the future education and training of nurses. The final report from the Shape of Caring review, *Raising the Bar* (2015), argued that more needed to be expected from future graduate nurses and recommended that greater acquisition of skills, previously considered advanced or post-registration, should be included in pre-registration programmes. This included the routine application of research evidence and innovation. The review also called for more nurse-led research to ensure evidence-based practice becomes more embedded, which in turn will improve quality of care. To do this, nurses need the knowledge and analytical skills to make informed decisions and contribute effectively to new innovations, taking a more proactive role in service improvement change and change management. The importance of research at pre-registration level is also acknowledged in the NMC outcomes (Nursing and Midwifery Council, 2018b), which reflect the proficiencies for accountable professional practice that must be applied across the standards of proficiency for registered nurses, and which explicitly state that newly qualified nurses must 'demonstrate an understanding of research methods, ethics and governance in order to critically analyse, safely use, share and apply research findings to promote and inform best nursing practice' (Nursing and Midwifery Council, 2018a: 5).

As a result of the above policy drivers, undergraduate nursing programmes are now required to provide education in research and students are expected to be consumers of research on qualifying.

There are calls for increasing numbers of nurses to undertake Master's and Doctoral level study, and exposure to research experience during undergraduate training as well as the utilisation of research in clinical practice can only support this ambition. Indeed, increasing numbers of registered nurses are engaging with research and, more importantly, seeking to implement research findings to underpin daily work (HEE, 2015). However, this is not seen as the norm and applies particularly to early-career nurses.

Increasingly, nurses and other healthcare professionals are taking on extended roles (previously the remit of the medical profession) requiring changes in their skillset and knowledge. Nurses need to acquire a strong grounding to develop a questioning approach to care that encourages them to challenge inappropriate care practice and to adopt an adaptive and innovative approach to care that seeks to impact positively on patient care experience. There are opportunities for academic staff to gain higher-level clinical and academic qualifications and indeed this is now a requirement for all healthcare academics. Although these roles make a vital contribution to evidence-based care, the number of clinical academics in nursing, midwifery and the allied health professions is less than 0.1% of the workforce. By contrast, clinical academics make up around 4.6% of the medical consultant workforce of the UK (Baltruks and Callaghan, 2018).

While the benefits of undergraduate education are recognised for both students and academic staff, it is important to discuss concerns around the transition from hospital-based schools to the higher education sector.

The transition to degree-level qualification from diploma necessitated, for most training establishments, a geographical relocation into a local higher education institution (HEI). The relocation of the schools to HEIs placed an additional burden on both clinicians and academic staff in terms of distance and, therefore, travelling times to meetings and supporting students in practice. Geographical isolation affects the ease with which healthcare professionals across the sectors interact and, therefore, maintain effective communication. In addition to this, many clinicians were concerned that provision of a graduate education would impact negatively on the clinical aspects of training and there was a concern that graduating students would be less clinically competent than their diplomate predecessors. These concerns were recognised by academic healthcare staff and there are systems in place to address these concerns. All undergraduate healthcare programmes are required to ensure that graduating students undertake a minimum number of hours of supervised and assessed clinical practice. Students are required to pass the clinical component prior to admission to the requisite professional register. There is a strong drive for theoretical components of programmes, including research modules, to be grounded in clinical practice. In order to better support this, clinicians are asked to support students by giving clinically relevant lectures, with some clinicians being offered honorary contracts with HEIs. Many HEIs now have clinical skills laboratories where students gain valuable clinical training skills relevant to their specific profession.

Healthcare academic staff who were part of the reforms seen in the 1980s and 1990s had to make adjustments to their professional development when the transfer to HEIs took place. The new profile for academic healthcare staff brings new tensions relating to their diverse responsibilities and accountabilities. They have had to gain academic qualifications (Bachelor degree through to PhD) to add to their professional curriculum vitae, integrate into a very different educational environment and support students undertaking new programmes. In addition to this, there are pressures on all academic staff to undertake and publish research in order to be recognised in the Research Exercise Framework (the formal system for assessing the quality of research in UK higher education institutions).

This period of transition for the academic healthcare workforce was for some academic staff an opportunity to develop their wider ambitions and move into leadership positions outside of their professional area. During the 1990s, new professorial positions were created, and appointments of deans of faculties and heads of college drawn from within the healthcare professions. Despite these notable leadership appointments, there was no coherent strategy to support career pathways development for healthcare academics recently repositioned into HEIs. At the same time, the schools of nursing, midwifery and allied professions received assistance from colleagues from NHS organisations in terms of offering specialist clinical teaching sessions and collaborative leadership support. Healthcare professionals from HEIs and the NHS could see that working effectively together by sharing expertise could bring mutual benefits to both communities and undergraduate students.

Local initiatives were developed across the four UK countries, with joint appointments created between trusts and HEIs and there was an emerging interest from clinical staff to undertake academic qualifications to support their continuing professional development. However, these achievements and collaborative arrangements were taking place without any direct and targeted support at a national level. Experienced clinicians attracted to a part-time role within a local HEI, found that differing pay scales and pension providers were barriers to developing a clinical academic career. HEIs were not able to match the salaries paid to experienced clinicians. There were problems with attempting to put together, for example, an honorary contract to allow clinicians to work in the education sector. Difficulties of coordinating activity across the health and educational sectors are still visible today and, more recently, recommendations have been made around defined working arrangements, with specific reference to developing and sustaining clinical academic careers. These are discussed further below.

Activity 11.3

Read the case studies below from two health professionals embarking on their clinical academic careers. Reflect on the relative benefits for both health and educational organisations.

Case study 11.2

'In a clinical academic career, I think you can have the best of both worlds. You can be in practice but also have the research skills to either drive research and evidence-based practice in your area, or be part of it.'
                              Nurse, Pre-PhD training programme participant

Case study 11.3

'I don't see myself as a clinical academic yet: I'm in the process of starting that journey. That's where I want to end up, but I am not quite there yet. ... I have learnt about my own qualities that I didn't know were there. It has made me feel up to date in my current area of practice by just having a chance to read and reflect. I'm more confident in my everyday interactions, taking on different things and approaching things with less doubt. I know that I have got involved with more research in my clinical area ... I have been involved in national research groups and attended more research events. This has made me more aware of what research is happening in the trust. I am more interested in reading around what is going on and bringing things that I find interesting to team meetings. I hear what's going on in the wider world of things: the courses I can go on, what's happening both nationally and in my local area. It has given me a new passion for what I am doing. Due to this, I had the confidence and motivation to set up my own journal group; we now have that culture where we are looking at new ideas and challenging what is going on. There has never been anyone to carry that through but now I've taken on that challenge and have the confidence to give it a go and see what comes from it.'

Nurse, Pre-PhD training programme participant

EARLY DEVELOPMENT OF INFRASTRUCTURE FOR CLINICAL ACADEMIC CAREERS

In 2003, the then Department of Health and the Department for Education and Skills, through its joint Strategic Learning and Research Advisory Group, commissioned a Project team led by Professor Tony Butterworth, then the Chief Executive of the Trent Workforce Confederation, to develop a Human Resources Plan to support educators and researchers across health and social care in the UK. National stakeholder consultations were undertaken and, in 2004, a Strategic Report (StLaR HR Plan Project Phase II Strategic Report) was published (Butterworth et al., 2004). The report made 15 recommendations, which are summarised collectively below:

- Develop flexible clinical academic employment models with pre-approved employment contracts together with transparent and accessible guidance relating to employment rights and pension transfer across the 'public sector pensions club'.
- Adopt key proposals from the Follett Review (2001) for medicine and dentistry where an individual retains a single key employer with joint appraisal and job planning mechanisms.
- Support consultant and advanced practitioners to fulfil their full obligations towards education and research, and support managers to work with their employees to consider flexible career options in education and research.
- For clinical trainees in medicine and dentistry, create a specific training pathway, which recognises the academic component through the National Training Number (NTN) Academic scheme.
- Improve the labour market intelligence system to provide accurate data on the disposition of the research and educator workforce for health and social care.

This report was presented to and received by the joint Strategic Learning and Research Advisory Group in 2004. It was agreed that further work should take place in order to build and expand on its recommendations.

In 2005, Sir Mark Walport was commissioned by the Department of Health to make recommendations for the future training of researchers and educators in medicine. This included creating a range of clinical academic training programmes in medicine. The report was written within the context of the UK but it was acknowledged that each of the four countries may wish to adapt the recommendations.

In nursing, the UK Clinical Research Collaboration (UKCRC) tasked Professor Tony Butterworth and Dr Christine Jackson (authors of the StLaR Plan Phase II Strategic Report) to develop the StLaR HR Plan further with a series of recommendations. This resulted in the publication of the 'Finch' Report (UKCRC, 2007), which was later adopted by the Modernising Nursing Careers initiative and was supported by the Chief Nursing Officers across the four countries within the UK. Although the title of the report reflects an initial remit to develop recommendations for the nursing profession, it was always the intention of the authors to include midwifery and allied health professions within the funding processes supporting these recommendations. The central and underlying principle of the recommendations was a vision for a flexible career pathway which places at its core a continued clinical career which is supported through targeted research training from Master's-level degree programmes, such as the Master's in Clinical Research, through to pre-professorial specialist research training.

The recommendations addressed three main areas: education and training, facilitating careers and better information. In relation to education and training, a progressive pathway was recommended to support clinical academic staff to progress though the various levels of a clinical academic career. Awards were recommended at different levels with, for example, first-level awards intended to support early-career healthcare professionals wishing to develop their clinical research skills through a defined research Master's programme, right through to higher-level awards intended to support post-doctoral clinical academics and prepare them for professorial and leadership positions.

In relation to facilitating careers, recommendations were made around supporting career flexibility to encourage rather than hinder careers which bridge both health and education sectors. They were based around the development of a model contract of employment for clinicians to take up research and academic roles without detrimental effects to salary and pension status and to find creative solutions, such as the use of honorary contracts in addition to substantive contracts with clearly defined and agreed roles, timeframes and appraisal systems. The report also acknowledged the importance of good mentorship in the support of aspiring clinical academics and those in more senior positions too. In medicine, there is a long-established tradition of appointing mentors to recipients of the equivalent awards in medicine. The Academy of Medical Sciences (AMS) supports all awardees in medicine through the management of the mentoring processes. The mentoring scheme is regarded as one of the crucial factors in the success of the training programmes, and establishing an equivalent mentoring scheme for healthcare professions was considered to be vital for the success of clinical academic training initiatives.

With regard to better information on nurse researchers, the recommendations for this section of the report related to promoting clinical academic careers to students on undergraduate programmes, healthcare managers and policy makers at local and regional levels.

Activity 11.4

Read the case studies below, which are extracts from interviews with health professionals who had recently embarked on a pre-Master's or a pre-PhD level clinical academic training programme. Reflect on the extent to which exposure to the training has already started to impact on the outlook and confidence levels of these clinicians and how evidence for changing practice is emerging.

'Being on the clinical academic pathway has made me recognise the skills I have got and the potential for those skills. There are a lot of really exciting opportunities to do something different and really make an impact. It [the training] gives you time out of the clinical workspace to consider where you want to go. I think it makes you more critical about what you do in practice, and why all the questioning and enquiring and being critical changes you as a person. My outlook is different now. I think it's about identifying what the issues are and being able to do something about them. I've been able to suggest to my managers ... "let's do a project". In previous years, I might not have had the skills or the confidence to say, "I've got these skills and I can use them ... let me put a project plan together, show you what the potential is". I can now recognise the value of these skills and highlight how they should be valued by the organisation in which I work. Whenever you learn something new, that changes your practice.'

Nurse, Pre-Master's programme participant

Case study 11.4

'A clinical academic career gives you the opportunity to contribute academically to your clinical role. I was looking for a different direction and the role was re-animating and re-energising. It has given me the opportunity to stand back and take a broader perspective of my clinical and professional life; and the direction I wanted it to go in. The role has increased my confidence in decision making but also my sense of achievement and motivation to achieve. I am now more inclined to take part in research as a clinician because I realise how difficult it is to get people to contribute to your research. I realise there is a lot out there still to learn, and that has elevated me a little bit and piqued my interest more. My confidence in being able to judge other people's assertions, with regard to research and new ideas, has increased considerably; and now I don't take things on face value quite so much, I mostly check things for myself.'

Paramedic, Pre-PhD programme participant

Case study 11.5

'A clinical academic career is about being clinically aware of research and being able to access information that could inform practice and help to move practice on. I think you have to be responsible for yourself in your practice. If you say as a nurse that you are evidence based in your practice, then you have to have some time to actually explore that. I didn't initially see myself as an academic as I hadn't really done much research. I wouldn't have attended research forums or conferences as I wouldn't have thought it was for me. Now I will go and I will expect to come away with something that will help my practice or that I can pass on.'

Nurse, Pre-Master's programme participant

Case study 11.6

Case study 11.7

'The role has given me more confidence to feel like I could make a difference, to want to make changes and to want to influence practice, but also, to make my own judgements. I wouldn't have had the confidence to be as challenging if I hadn't gone through the process of having two papers published; doing the research, being confident in my practice and in how I was delivering things. I think it's also about the confidence and the knowledge of where to go with what I don't know. I've built a network of people that I can tap into, my behaviour of resourcing and sharing has made an impact on how my clinical team perform. There are national guidelines and tools that some of the people in the team didn't even know about. I am now able to share that knowledge.'

Nurse, Pre-Master's programme participant

CURRENT PROVISION

The reports described above brought clinical academic careers onto the political agenda and paved the way for tangible developments and the beginning of opportunities for health professionals wishing to pursue a clinical academic career. Fellowships to support the training and development of early-career clinical academics are now offered by a range of funders. The report *Developing the Best Research Professionals* (UKCRC, 2007) led to the establishment of a national Clinical Academic Training (CAT) programme. By promoting a partnership between universities and healthcare providers, in England support for clinical academic careers is now starting to become established, and government-funded training to gain recognised qualifications, such as a Master's degree or a PhD, is now well established. The NIHR/HEE now fund a clinical academic pathway, which provides a range of academic opportunities, from internships through to postgraduate and post-doctoral education to professorships. A fundamental priority of this programme is the 'integrated' approach that emphasises both clinical and academic input into creating new collaborative posts between a hospital NHS Trust and an academic institution (HEE, 2014). Opportunities have also been developed in Scotland (NHS Education for Scotland, 2010) and Ireland.

A key recommendation from the Shape of Caring report (HEE, 2015) was the development of Doctoral Training Centres (DTCs), which support clinical registered nurses academically, and encourage an increase in active 'on-the-ground' research within a sound support structure while providing a clear academic pathway. It was also recommended that registered nurses who choose to complete a thesis or Quality Improvement Project as part of a post-qualification preceptorship programme could regard these as an initial stage of research training that could later enable them to apply to study for a postgraduate research degree (such as a Master's or PhD), in an area that makes a direct difference to frontline patient care. In response, doctoral training schools, open to nurses, midwives and allied health professionals, began to emerge across the UK.

Health Education England (HEE) has a statutory responsibility to promote research. The Health and Social Care Act 2012, HEE Directions 2013 and the Mandate from the Government to HEE, require HEE to 'develop a more flexible workforce that is able to respond to the changing patterns of service and embraces research and innovation to enable it to adapt to the changing demands of public health, healthcare and care services (DH, 2014: 29). HEE also has a statutory responsibility and mandate to undertake the development of a transparent and integrated multi-professional clinical academic career framework, which enables all partners to be clear about the strategic approach to developing the clinical academic workforce for patient benefit, and a specific objective to 'support clinical academic careers for health professionals and also seek to increase numbers of staff across all clinical and public health professions with a proper understanding of research and its role in improving health outcomes, including an ability to participate in and utilise the result of research' (DH, 2014: 30). Indeed, integrated infrastructure across the health and educational sectors is key to the success and sustainability of clinical academic careers for individual practitioners, as they cannot happen in isolation. The national strategy for their development emphasises the role and importance of leadership in clinical teams so it is essential that clinical academics are equipped with the skills needed to examine the optimal characteristics of the workplace environment such that they can influence colleagues to foster the development of a research culture in their own clinical setting. This should include discussion of how to maximise input from those in different professional or clinical settings and how to influence others to adopt an inclusive approach across the wider clinical arena, incorporating multidisciplinary staff.

Barriers to successful implementation of training programmes for clinical academics have been identified (such as the competing immediate and longer-term demands faced by managers in the clinical setting). In acknowledgement of this, a number of initiatives have been put in place to support managers in the support of others. For example, a toolkit for NHS managers to provide support for clinical practice in the development of clinical academic careers has been published by AUKUH (www.medschools.ac.uk/media/2325/aukuh-transforming-healthcare.pdf) as well as a handbook from NIHR, published as a negotiating prop through which aspiring clinical academics can begin difficult conversations (National Institute for Health Research, 2016).

It has been acknowledged (Willis Commission, 2012) that employers need to recognise the evidence regarding the benefits and return on investment of nursing, midwifery and allied health professional leaders who successfully combine practical clinical and academic work. Transforming the partnership between health and higher education requires a commitment to growing and developing clinical academic practice from within the current workforce.

Summary

- Educational programmes for registered nurses, midwives and allied health professionals are largely delivered at least at degree level or are moving towards doing so.
- There is increasing emphasis on the importance of content relating to research, including the generation, critique and implementation of evidence-based practice in pre-registration educational programmes.

(Continued)

- Opportunities for the development of clinical academic careers have been emerging for some years in the UK and elsewhere and are now becoming more readily available.
- The benefits of supporting health professionals to develop their research skills and experience while remaining as active clinicians have been established.
- Good collaborative working relationships between the health and educational sectors are crucial to the success of clinical academic career initiatives.

FURTHER READING

AUKUH Clinical Academic Roles Development Group (2017) *Transforming healthcare through clinical academic roles in nursing, midwifery and allied health professions.* www.medschools.ac.uk/media/2325/aukuh-transforming-healthcare.pdf

Baltruks, D. and Callaghan, P. (2018) *Nursing, Midwifery and Allied Health Clinical Academic Research Careers in the UK.* Council of Deans of Health, August. https://councilofdeans.org.uk/wp-content/uploads/2018/08/Nursing-midwifery-and-allied-health-clinical-academic-research-careers-in-the-UK.pdf

Council of Deans of Health (2020) Improving clinical academic careers for nurses, midwives and allied health professionals. Position Paper. March. https://councilofdeans.org.uk/wp-content/uploads/2020/09/13032020-CoDH-CAC-position-statement-draft-1.pdf

Council of Deans of Health (2019) *Becoming research confident: Research in pre-registration curricula for nursing, midwifery and allied health programmes in the UK.*

Council of Deans of Health (2018) *Nursing, midwifery and allied health clinical academic research careers in the UK.*

Council of Deans of Health (2017) *High performing research environments in nursing, midwifery and allied health professions.*

Department of Health (2012) *Developing the Role of the Clinical Academic Researcher in Nursing, Midwifery and the Allied Health Professions.* London: Department of Health.

Medical Research Council (2015) *A cross-funder review of early-career clinical academics: Enablers and barriers to progression.* A review led by the Medical Research Council in collaboration with the Academy of Medical Sciences, British Heart Foundation, Cancer Research UK, National Institute for Health Research and Wellcome Trust. www.mrc.ukri.org/documents/pdf/review-of-early-career-clinical-academics/

NIHR (2019) *Research in the NHS – HR good practice resource pack.* www.myresearchproject.org.uk/help/hlphrgoodpractice.aspx

United Kingdom Clinical Research Collaboration (2007) *Clinical Academic Careers for Nurses, Midwives and Allied Health Professionals.* London: UKCRC.

United Kingdom Clinical Research Collaboration Subcommittee for Nurses in Clinical Research (Workforce) (2007) *Developing the Best Research Professionals: Qualified Graduate Nurses: Recommendations for Preparing and Supporting Clinical Academic Nurses of the Future: The 'Finch' Report.* London: UKCRC.

USEFUL WEBLINKS

Academic Science Health Networks (AHSN): a network of 15 Academic Health Science Networks (AHSNs) was established by NHS England in 2013 to spread innovation – improving health and generating economic growth. Each AHSN works across a distinct geography serving a different population in each region. www.ahsnnetwork.com

The University Hospital Association (UHA): the key leadership body across the UK promoting the tripartite interests of university hospitals: service, teaching and research. Its role is to represent University Hospital Trusts' unique interests in partnership with other national bodies. www.university hospitals.org.uk/

Applied Research Collaborations (ARCs) are funded by the National Institute for Health Research and support applied health and care research across England. www.nihr.ac.uk/explore-nihr/support/collaborating-in-applied-health-research.htm

The Council of Deans of Health (CoD): represents the UK's university faculties engaged in education and research for nurses, midwives and allied health professionals. It operates as a multiprofessional organisation at the heart of policy and political debate, and aims to lead policy at national and UK level and for some years has identified the development and support for clinical academic careers as a priority. Many relevant documents pertaining to this topic are published and available via their website: www.councilofdeans.org.uk

The Health and Care Professions Council (HCPC): the independent regulating body for health, psychological and social work professionals in the UK. www.hcpc-uk.org

The National Institute of Health Research (NIHR): funds health research and aims to ensure that the NHS is able to support the research of other funders to encourage broader investment in, and economic growth from, health research. Specifically the NIHR funds clinical academic trainingpathways.www.nihr.ac.uk/explore-nihr/academy-programmes/hee-nihr-integrated-clinical-academic-programme.htm

NIHR Evidence, funded by the National Institute of Health Research in England aims to make health and care research findings informative, accessible, relevant and readily available. NIHR Evidence presents high quality summaries of findings so that health and care research can be used by everyone. https://evidence.nihr.ac.uk

The UK Clinical Research Collaboration (UKCRC): a forum which promotes a strategic approach to the identification of opportunities and obstacles to clinical research and aims to establish a network to enable people to work together to transform the clinical research environment in the UK. www.ukcrc.org

UK Research and Innovation (UKRI): invests in close collaboration with others to build a thriving, inclusive research and innovation system. www.ukri.org

Vitae is a global leader in supporting the professional development of researchers, experienced in working with institutions as they strive for research excellence, innovation and impact. They have published a very useful and widely used framework to support and direct research career development which is freely available: www.vitae.ac.uk/doing-research/leadership-development-for-principal-investigators-pis/developing-individual-researchers/supporting-researcher-career-development

Conclusion to Part III

The aim of this section was to provide you with the necessary skills, knowledge and tools to enable you to make changes to your practice as appropriate and ensure your practice continues to be evidence-based throughout your career. Hopefully you have now:

- identified ways in which changes can be made to practice and issues you need to consider before making changes;
- considered how best to reflect on your experiences and used that reflection to enhance your practice;
- identified your needs in relation to lifelong learning;
- developed confidence in your ability to used evidence appropriately in the delivery of care.

This part ends with a crossword puzzle, with clues to words relevant to Chapters 9 and 10. The answers can be found on p. 220.

ACROSS

3. A cycle for improvement (4)

5. Those people who might have an interest in something (11)

7. Restoration or renewal (10)

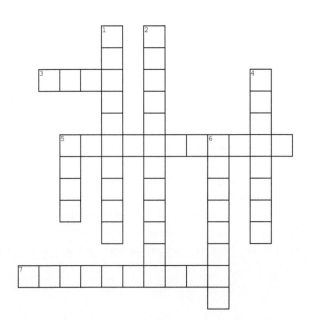

DOWN

1. Making a judgement of something (10)
2. Someone who facilitates change in practice (6,5)
4. A quality improvement process (8)
5. A type of analysis that allows for personal development (4)
6. Learning aimed at ensuring knowledge/skills are up-to-date (8)

Appendices

Appendix 1
Template for Decision Aid

Date prepared ....

Name of intervention	
Aim of decision aid	
Description: (mode of delivery, frequency, restriction)	
How does it work?	
Extent of effectiveness	
Goal to be achieved	
What will be required of the patient?	
Benefits	
Risks	
Side effects	
Effect on quality of life	
Sources of further information	
References	
Other options (it may be necessary to prepare individual sheets for each option)	

Appendix 2

Formulating a Question and Searching for Evidence

1. Define your topic

What is your area of interest?

Break down your topic into key concepts using the PICO formula to create a clear clinical question:

Patient/problem	Intervention	Comparison	Outcome(s)

What is your question?

2. Define your scope/limits

Date range:

Language:

Type of studies:

Other:

3. Identify relevant resources to search

Appropriate databases to search:

4. Identify search terms

Consider any alternative terms/spellings, abbreviations, acronyms, etc. for your PICO concepts and list below:

Patient/problem	Intervention	Comparison	Outcome(s)

Check your selected databases for appropriate subject headings and include them in the table above. This information can then be used to build your search strategy. You can combine search terms together by using the Boolean operators 'AND', 'OR' and 'NOT'.

5. Undertake your search and evaluate the results

Reflection on this learning experience:

Action(s) to be taken:

Appendix 3

General Critical Appraisal Tool for Research Studies

Section	Things to consider
Title	• Does it clearly identify the area of study?
Abstract	• Does it contain enough information for you to decide whether or not the paper is of interest to you?
Authors' qualifications	• Are these appropriate for the area of study?
Introduction	• Does it clearly outline the area of interest and give a rationale for the paper? • Is the research question and/or hypothesis clearly identified? • Is a theoretical/conceptual framework identified?
Literature review	• Is there a critical review of the literature related to the area of study? • Is the literature appropriate, up to date, mainly from primary sources, and does it include any seminal works associated with the topic?
Conceptual/ theoretical framework	• Are concepts clearly defined? • Is there a fit between the conceptual framework and the research design?
Ethical issues	• Has ethical approval been acquired? • Are the potential risks and benefits discussed? • Are sources of funding and outside interests identified?
Design	• Is the design clearly stated/described allowing for replication? • Is it appropriate to the study? • Are the strengths and limitations debated?
Methodology	• Is this appropriate to the research question/hypothesis and aims of the study? • How are the data to be collected? • What sampling methods are used and are these appropriate to the methodology? • Are issues of reliability, validity, trustworthiness and rigour considered?

Section	Things to consider
Results	• Does it give a clear description of how the results were reached? • Are the results clearly described and presented in a way that promotes understanding?
Discussion	• Are all the results explored and explained? • Is there consistency between the results and the arguments put forward? • Are the arguments logically developed and do they take account of opposing views? • Is the interpretation offered reasonable and does it make sense in light of what you know about the subject area?
Conclusions	• Are these logical and coherent? • Do these 'fit' with the data and the arguments presented in the discussion?
Recommendations/ limitations	• Are these presented in a clear way? • Is there a logical link between the findings and the recommendation?
Applicability to practice	• Is the sample used similar to the patients/service users in your area of practice? • Is training required to implement the findings? • Are considerations such as costs accounted for? • Do the benefits of changing practice outweigh any identified harmful effects?

Appendix 4
Critical Appraisal Tool for Quantitative Research Studies

Area	Issues for consideration
Hypotheses/research questions	• Are the research questions and/or hypotheses clear, unambiguous and where appropriate capable of being tested? • Are these consistent with the conceptual framework and research design?
Literature review	• Is there a critical review of the literature related to the area of study? • Is the literature appropriate, up to date, mainly from primary sources, and including any seminal works associated with the topic?
Conceptual/theoretical framework	• Are the concepts clearly defined? • Is there a fit between the conceptual framework and the research design?
Operational definitions	• Are all terms used clearly defined? • Does it identify how variables will be observed and measured?
Design	• Is the design clearly stated/described allowing for replication? • Is it appropriate to the study? • Are issues which may result in bias minimised? • Are the strengths and limitations debated?
Data collection methods	• Are these adequately described? • Are the instruments adequately described and appropriate to the study's purpose and design? • Are the instruments used valid, reliable and reproducible?

Area	Issues for consideration
Sampling method	• Is the population of interest identified? • Are the subject characteristics clearly identified? • Are the inclusion and exclusion criteria clearly identified and appropriate? • Is the sampling approach appropriate to the design? • Is the size of sample identified and adequate? • Are power calculations present where appropriate?
Ethical issues	• Has ethical approval been acquired? • Are the potential risks and benefits discussed? • Are sources of funding and outside interests identified?
Data analysis	• Is it appropriate to the type of data? • Is complete information reported? • Is there adequate description of any subjects who were withdrawn from the study?
Findings	• Are these presented in a clear and understandable way? • Do tables/charts make sense? • Are data described in sufficient detail?
Discussion	• Is it balanced, including all major findings? • Are results considered in light of other research? • Does it address issues of generalisability? • Is there an acknowledgement of limitation?
Validity, reliability, applicability	• Are the results valid and reliable? • Is the relevance for practice identified?

Appendix 5

Critical Appraisal Tool for Qualitative Research Studies

Area	Issues for consideration
Research question and aims	• Is the question clearly stated and appropriate to the topic area? • Are the aims clearly stated and relevant to the research question?
Literature review	• Is there a critical review of the literature related to the area of study? • Is the literature appropriate, up to date, mainly from primary sources, and including any seminal works associated with the topic?
Conceptual/theoretical framework	• Are concepts clearly defined? • Is there a fit between the conceptual framework and the research design?
Design	• Is the design clearly stated/described, allowing for replication? • Is it appropriate to the study? • Are the strengths and limitations debated?
Methodology	• Is a qualitative approach appropriate? • Is a specific approach used and described? • Does the research give a clear justification for the research design?
Reflexivity	• Does the researcher(s) provide a statement identifying their position/perspective?
Ethical issues	• Has ethical approval been acquired? • Are the potential risks and benefits discussed? • Are sources of funding and outside interests identified?
Sampling/participants	• Is the sampling method appropriate and clearly described?

Area	Issues for consideration
Data collection	• Are the data collection methods appropriate to the research approach and design? • Are the methods described in enough detail for you to understand the process?
Data analysis	• Is the data analysis tool identified and appropriate to the type of data and research design?
Findings	• Are the findings presented in a clear way? • Is there sufficient information to understand how the findings were reached? • Are the findings credible? • Are these discussed in light of other research/literature? • Are the study's limitations identified?
Conclusions	• Are these logical and coherent? • Do these 'fit' with the data presented and the arguments presented in the discussion?
Issues of rigour	• Have steps been taken to ensure the findings have credibility, transferability, dependability, confirmability and authenticity?
Applicability to practice	• Is the sample used similar to the patients/service users in your area of practice? • Is training required to implement the findings? • Are considerations such as costs accounted for? • Do the benefits of changing practice outweigh any identified harmful effects?

Appendix 6
Critical Appraisal Tool for Systematic Reviews

Area	Issues for consideration
Question	• Is there a clear and precisely defined question? • Are all terms/concepts clearly defined? • Are the inclusion and exclusion criteria clearly identified?
Search strategy	• What search terms were identified to search for studies, were these appropriate/exhaustive? • What databases were searched and were these appropriate? • Was a thorough search of all sources of literature undertaken, including grey literature?
Quality appraisal	• How was the quality of the studies assessed? • Is a checklist/tool identified for critical appraisal? • Did two or more reviewers appraise the literature? • Did the reviewers provide a rationale for exclusion of any studies?
Data extraction	• Has information about sample characteristics been extracted? • Is there sufficient information about the findings?
Summarising the evidence	• Where meta-analysis/synthesis is not used is this adequately justified? • Are the methods of 'pooling' data clearly explained? • Is the data analysis thorough and credible?
Meta-analysis	• Were two or more reviewers involved in the data extraction, ensuring the integrity of the data set? • Are treatment effects reported for all relevant outcomes? • How large is the treatment effect? • Is the heterogeneity of treatment effects adequately addressed?

Area	Issues for consideration
Meta-synthesis	<ul><li>Were two or more reviewers involved in the data extraction, ensuring the integrity of the data set?</li><li>Is a fuller understanding of the phenomenon of interest achieved?</li><li>Are the interpretations appropriate and sound?</li><li>Are examples of data provided to support interpretations?</li></ul>
Conclusions	<ul><li>Are these coherent and do they flow from the findings?</li><li>Is the strength of the evidence discussed?</li></ul>
Recommendations/ limitations	<ul><li>What recommendations are made?</li><li>Are potential limitations identified?</li></ul>
Applicability to practice	<ul><li>Are implications for practice explored?</li><li>How similar is the population of the studies to the patient group you are interested in?</li></ul>

Appendix 7
Action Planning

Goal: *What do I want to achieve?*
Rationale: *Why?*
Action: *How will I go about it?*
Criteria for success: *How will I know when I've got there?*
Evaluation: *What have I achieved and what next?*

Appendix 8
Personal Development Plan

What do I want to achieve? (goals)	How will this help my personal development?	How will I achieve it?	What help do I need?
1.			
2.			
3.			
Evaluation:			

Appendix 9

Summary Table of Study Details

Study details (full reference)	Pre-appraised evidence (Yes/No level 1–6)*	Study design (methodology and method)	Intervention/ phenomenon of interest	Setting (e.g. hosp/ community), geographical location, e.g. UK	Participants/ subjects (number, age, gender, ethnicity, cultural context)	Type of data analysis	Key findings	Quality	Applicability to practice

*Pre-appraised data hierarchy (DiCenso et al., 2013):

1. Systems
2. Summaries
3. Synopses of syntheses
4. Syntheses
5. Synopses of single studies
6. Critically appraised individual studies

Appendix 10
SWOT Analysis

Strengths *What are my strengths?* *What am I good at?*	**Weaknesses** *What are my current limitations?* *What might I do/think that would stop me meeting my goal?*
Opportunities *What will help in achieving my goal?* *What resources are available to me?*	**Threats** *What barriers are there to me achieving my goal - personal and organisational?*

Solutions to Word Puzzles

SOLUTION TO PART I CROSSWORD

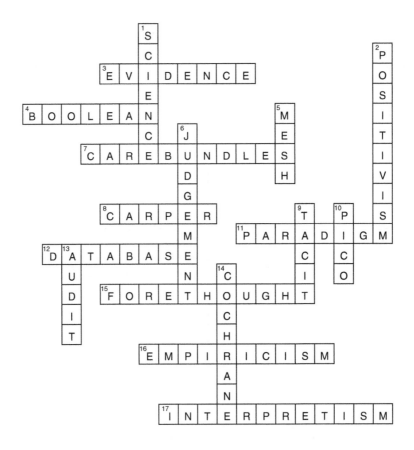

SOLUTION TO PART II WORD SEARCH

Hidden words:

Validity; reliability; trustworthiness; credibility; dependability; comfirmability; transferability; rigour; variable; hypothesis; probability; stratified; bracketing; meta-analysis; randomised; trial; snowball; mean; mode; emic; etic

J	T	R	I	A	L	U	O	U	T	Q	T	V	Q	U	X	T	E	V	X
A	G	M	U	Q	V	A	R	I	A	B	L	E	S	E	L	R	O	E	D
S	K	S	Q	Q	L	X	R	I	G	O	U	R	E	B	H	U	M	G	H
K	V	S	J	R	S	J	C	F	D	N	B	T	Y	T	N	S	N	Z	S
K	W	Y	B	F	N	K	O	Q	A	P	F	B	E	R	Z	T	J	R	T
M	A	Z	R	T	O	Q	N	N	Z	R	E	J	U	A	Z	W	D	A	R
O	V	H	A	T	W	E	F	Z	R	O	Z	F	I	N	Y	O	E	N	A
D	S	Y	C	D	B	Y	I	X	E	B	U	F	J	S	H	R	P	D	T
E	M	P	K	W	A	R	R	K	L	A	P	E	Q	F	F	T	E	O	I
R	E	O	E	A	L	E	M	E	I	B	T	T	L	E	F	H	N	M	F
Y	T	T	T	J	L	D	A	F	A	I	K	I	A	R	E	I	D	I	I
A	A	H	I	L	R	V	B	X	B	L	D	C	L	A	W	N	A	S	E
K	A	E	N	D	E	O	I	G	I	I	G	D	N	B	Z	E	B	E	D
E	N	S	G	I	Q	B	L	E	L	T	U	U	L	I	W	S	I	D	S
U	A	I	T	U	R	K	I	E	I	Y	F	G	K	L	Z	S	L	O	S
N	L	S	T	V	P	B	T	Z	T	F	F	Z	U	I	V	E	I	A	B
K	Y	C	W	R	W	J	Y	A	Y	M	E	A	N	T	K	R	T	C	P
L	S	U	J	E	M	I	C	B	A	S	N	K	M	Y	V	W	Y	G	O
S	I	U	F	R	T	Z	Y	P	R	I	V	A	L	I	D	I	T	Y	T
C	S	K	C	R	E	D	I	B	I	L	I	T	Y	T	D	F	R	C	B

SOLUTION TO PART III CROSSWORD

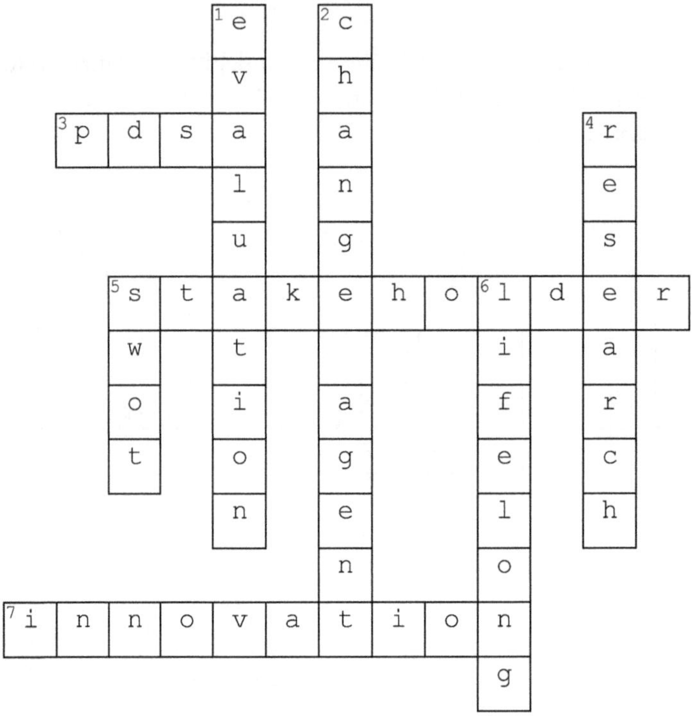
1 evaluation
2 change agent
3 pdsa
4 research
5 stakeholder
swot
6 lifelong
7 innovation

Glossary of Terms

A priori   knowledge arrived at through reasoning processes.

Authority   knowledge coming from a source or person viewed as being authoritative.

Background question   generally a broad who, what, where, when, how, why question about an area of clinical interest.

Bracketing   a process used in qualitative research, where one's own thoughts and feelings in relation to the study are acknowledged and then 'placed on one side' to allow an unbiased analysis of the data.

Care bundles   three to five items of practice evidence grouped together in relation to a particular condition, treatment and/or procedure which have a more positive impact on treatment outcomes than any one single element.

Change agent   someone who facilitates change in the practice setting using specific interventions to implement and evaluate evidence-based practices.

Change management   the process of promoting change through the use of specific management theories and approaches.

Citation pearl growing   a way of identifying literature of interest by using an initial article (pearl) of interest to identify appropriate subject headings.

Clinical audit   an approach whereby clinical practices are measured against agreed explicit standards to promote clinical effectiveness.

Clinical effectiveness   the delivery of care in the most appropriate and evidence-based way.

Clinical governance   the process and structures put in place within healthcare institutions to promote and maintain quality of care.

Confirmability   the process of creating an audit trail of decisions taken in relation to analysis of qualitative data.

Correlation studies   quantitative research approach which examines relationships between variables without manipulation of the independent variable.

Credibility   processes put in place to ensure the findings of qualitative research are seen to be appropriate and representing the participants' experiences.

Critical appraisal   a careful evaluation of the worth, value or quality of evidence.

Cross-sectional studies   research which compares different groups within a population of interest, collecting data at a single identified point in time.

Data saturation   a term used in grounded theory research to indicate the point where no new information is being generated during the collection of data through the use of interviews.

Deductive reasoning   reasoning which moves from general theories to a specific hypothesis.

Dependability   a term used in assessing the quality of qualitative research, identifying the need to ensure all participant perspectives are accounted for in the analysis of data and presentation of findings.

Descriptive studies   quantitative research which observes, describes and documents areas of interest as they occur naturally.

Disproportional sampling   a form of sampling used in quantitative research where a larger sample of a particular subgroup (e.g. age, ethnicity) is used than is present within a population, usually where there is a need to consider the relationship between variables in that group.

Empiricism   in philosophy, empiricism is a theory that states that knowledge comes only or primarily from sensory experience. Empiricism emphasises the role of empirical evidence in the formation of ideas, rather than innate ideas or traditions.

Evidence   an organised body of knowledge used to support or justify actions and beliefs.

Evidence-based medicine   an approach to the delivery of medical practice aimed at ensuring all activities are based on rigorous evidence.

Foreground question   a focused question formed in relation to a specific issue, looking for particular knowledge.

Grey literature   literature which has not been formally published, includes theses and/or dissertations, conference proceedings and in-house publications such as leaflets, newsletters and pamphlets.

Hermeneutics   related to meaning and interpretation – how people interpret their experiences within a specific context.

Hypothesis   a simple statement identifying a testable relationship between at least two clearly stated variables.

Idealism   the view that associates reality to ideas in the mind rather than to material objects.

Inductive reasoning   reasoning which flows from thoughts related to a particular issue to a general theory.

Interpretivism   an alternative to positivism based on the belief that humans are actively involved in constructing their understanding of the world.

Intuitive knowledge   a form of tacit knowledge, which involves arriving at conclusions without being aware of thinking in a rational and logical way to generate that knowledge.

Lifelong learning   self-directed learning in which the aim is to ensure that knowledge and skills remain up to date.

Longitudinal studies   research in which data are collected at various points over an extended period of time from an identified individual/group of people.

Materialism   the view that all facts are causally dependent upon physical processes.

MeSH terms   medical subject headings commonly used in certain databases to describe the contents of an article.

Meta-analysis   the pooling of data from a number of quantitative research studies to provide a larger data set.

Meta-synthesis   the pooling of findings from a number of qualitative research studies.

Mixed methodsrefers to an emergent methodology of research that advances the systematic integration, or 'mixing', of quantitative and qualitative data within a single investigation or sustained program of inquiry. ... Integrating the data during data collection, analysis, or discussion.

Non-propositional knowledgepersonal knowledge linked to experience that is used by individuals to help them think and act.

Paradigma collection of ideas and concepts providing a theoretical perspective on how knowledge can be generated through research.

Participantspeople who make up the sample in qualitative research.

PICO questionformat used to help to create a search question in relation to a particular clinical issue in which P = population; I = intervention; C = comparison; O = outcome.

Positivisma belief that reality is ordered, regular, and can be studied objectively and quantified.

Proportional stratified samplinga form of sampling used in quantitative research to ensure subgroups (e.g. by age, ethnicity) within a population are present in a sample in the same proportions.

Propositional knowledgepublic knowledge, usually given a formal status by its inclusion in educational programmes.

Prospective studieswhere data are collected in relation to a specific independent variable and the dependent variable is measured at a later date.

Publication biasthe tendency to publish studies that report positive results, resulting in a reported bias towards the effectiveness of a particular intervention.

Realismthe belief that objects continue to exist in the world even when no one is there to see them.

Reflectionthe process by which someone actively considers an experience, critically appraising it in light of experience and knowledge, and develops new perspectives to be tested in new situations.

Relevancea consideration as to whether the findings from a study can be applied to the practice setting.

Reliabilityconcerned with identifying if the results of a research study are dependable and replicable.

Retrospective studiesresearch in which data are collected after an event of interest. For example, patients' notes may be examined for information in relation to a specific treatment and recovery.

Rigourensuring that research is of high quality, conducted in an appropriate way, consistent with the underpinning philosophical principles.

Sampling unitspeople who form the sample within quantitative research, sometimes known as subjects.

Sciencea body of knowledge, based on observation, experiment and measurement, organised in a systematic manner.

Search enginean electronic device which enables you to search the World Wide Web for information.

Search strategyA search strategy is the information (keywords, subject headings, etc.) that you enter into a database to find relevant evidence.

Secondary researchresearch using data from primary research rather from an original source.

Service evaluation   a systematic approach to gaining insight into patient satisfaction with services.

Shared decision making   a partnership involving the sharing of information between at least two individuals (patient and health professional) to facilitate collaborative decision making.

Subjects   people who form the sample within quantitative research, sometimes known as sampling units.

Synthesis   a written discussion incorporating support from several sources of differing views.

Systematic review   a rigorous review of research findings in relation to a specific clinical question.

Tacit knowledge   knowledge well known to practitioners but not evident within the research-based literature.

Tenacity   a source of knowledge believed simply because it has always been held as the truth.

Transferability   a term used in qualitative research to describe the tentative application of research findings from one study to another, similar group of participants.

Triangulation   an approach used in qualitative research to increase the rigour of the findings. Entails considering the phenomenon of interest from different angles – usually in terms of its data, methodology, investigators, theoretical framework.

Trustworthiness   whether data from a research study can be considered dependable and credible.

Validity   whether or not the claims made in a research study are accurate.

Variables   are factors or traits that are likely to vary from one person/situation to another such as weight, temperature, pain, personality traits.

References

Aas, R. W. and Alexanderson, K. (2011) 'Challenging evidence-based decision-making: a hypothetical case study about return to work', *Occupational Therapy International*, 19: 28–44.

Acosta, S., Garza, T., Hsu, H.-Y. and Goodson, P. (2020) 'Assessing quality in systematic literature reviews: a study of novice rater training', *SAGE Open*, 10(3). https://doi.org/10.1177/2158244020939530

Akobeng, A.K. (2005) 'Understanding systematic reviews and meta-analysis', *Archives of Disease in Childhood*, 90(8): 845–8.

Alatawi, M., Aljuhani, E., Alsufiany, F., Aleid, K., Rawah, R., Aljanabi, S. and Banakhar, M. (2020) 'Barriers of implementing evidence-based practice in nursing profession: a literature review', *American Journal of Nursing Science*, 9(1): 35–42. doi: 10.11648/j.ajns.20200901.16.

Alkin, M. C. and Christie, C. A. (2004) 'An evaluation theory tree', in M. C. Alkin (ed.) *Evaluation Roots*. Thousand Oaks, CA: Sage. pp. 12-65.

Alper, B.S. and Haynes, R.B. (2016) 'EBHC pyramid 5.0 for accessing preappraised evidence and guidance', *Evidence Based Medicine*, 21(4): 123–5.

Anfara, V.A. Jr and Mertz, N.T. (2006) 'Conclusion: coming full circle', in V.A. Anfara Jr and N.T. Mertz (eds) *Theoretical Frameworks in Qualitative Research*. Thousand Oaks, CA: Sage. pp. 189–96.

Arcadi, P., Simonetti, V., Ambrosca, R., Cicolini, G., Simeone, S., Pucciarelli, G., Alvaro, R., Vellone, E. and Durante, A. (2021) 'Nursing during the COVID-19 outbreak: a phenomenological study', *Journal of Nursing Management*, 29(5): 1111–19.

Aromataris, E., Fernandez, R., Godfrey, C., Holly, C., Kahlil, H. and Tungpunkom, P. (2015) 'Summarizing systematic reviews: methodological development, conduct and reporting of an umbrella review approach', *International Journal of Evidence-Based Healthcare*, 13(3): 132–40.

Aspers, P. and Corte, U. (2019) 'What is qualitative in qualitative research', *Qualitative Sociology*, 42(2): 139–60. doi:10.1007/s11133-019-9413-7

Association of UK University Hospitals (AUKUH) (2016) *Transforming Healthcare through Clinical Academic Roles in Nursing, Midwifery and Allied Health Professions: A Practical Resource for Healthcare Provider Organisations*. AUKUH Clinical Academic Roles Development Group.

Azorin, J. and Cameron, R. (2010) 'The application of mixed methods in organisational research: a literature review', *Electronic Journal of Business Research Methods*, 8(2): 95–105.

Backhouse, A. and Ogunlayi, F. (2020) 'Quality improvement into practice', *BMJ*, 368: m865.

Baltruks, D. and Callaghan, P. (2018) *Nursing, Midwifery and Allied Health Clinical Academic Research Careers in the UK*. Council of Deans of Health, August.

Barkham, M. and Mellor-Clark, J. (2003) 'Bridging evidence-based practice and practice-based evidence: developing a rigorous and relevant knowledge for the psychological therapies', *Clinical Psychology and Psychotherapy*, 10: 319–27.

Barksby, J., Butcher, N. and Whysall, A. (2015) 'A new model of reflection for clinical practice', *Nursing Times*, 111(34–35): 21–3.

Behari-Leak, K. (2017) 'New academics, new higher education contexts: a critical perspective on professional development', *Teaching in Higher Education*, 22(5): 485–500.

Benner, P. (1984) *From Novice to Expert: Excellence and Power in Clinical Nursing Practice*. Menlo Park, CA: Addison Wesley.

Benner, P., Tanner, C. and Chelsea, C. (1996) *Expertise in Nursing Practice: Caring, Clinical Judgment, and Ethics*. New York: Springer.

Bergdahl, E. (2019) 'Is meta-aggregation a viable method for qualitative evidence synthesis? A reply to the commentary by Lockwood et al.', *Nursing Inquiry*, 26(4): e12325.

Bhaskar, R. (1975) *A Realist Theory of Science*. London: Verso.

Bhaskar, R. (1989) *Reclaiming Reality: A Critical Introduction to Contemporary Philosophy*. London: Verso.

Billay, D., Myrick, F., Luhanga, F. and Yonge, O. (2007) 'A pragmatic view of intuitive knowledge in nursing practice', *Nursing Forum*, 42(3): 147–55.

BMJ (2007) 'Medical milestones, celebrating key advances since 1840', *BMJ*, 334(suppl): s1–22.

Boaz, A., Hanney, S., Jones, T., et al. (2015) 'Does the engagement of clinicians and organisations in research improve healthcare performance: a three-stage review', *BMJ Open*, 5: e009415.

Booth, A. (2004) 'Formulating answerable questions', in A. Booth and A. Brice (eds) *Evidence Based Practice for Information Professionals: A Handbook*. London: Facet.

Booth, A. (2006) '"Brimful of STARLITE": toward standards for reporting literature searches', *Journal of the American Medical Library Association*, 94(4): 421-29.

Booth, A., Sutton, A. and Papaioannou, D. (2016a) *Systematic Approaches to a Successful Literature Review* (2nd edn). London: Sage.

Booth, A., Noyes, J., Flemming, K., Gerhardus, A., Wahlster, P., van der Wilt, G.J., Mozygemba, K., Refolo, P., Sacchini, D., Tummers, M. and Rehfuess, E. (2016b) *Guidance on choosing qualitative evidence synthesis methods for use in health technology assessments of complex interventions*. www.integrate-hta.eu/downloads/ [accessed 25 August 2021].

Boutron, I., Page, M.J., Higgins, J.P.T., Altman, D.G., Lundh, A. and Hróbjartsson, A. (2021) 'Considering bias and conflicts of interest among the included studies', in J.P.T. Higgins, J. Thomas, J. Chandler, M. Cumpston, T. Li, M.J. Page and V.A. Welch (eds) *Cochrane Handbook for Systematic Reviews of Interventions: version 6.2*. London: Cochrane. https://training.cochrane.org/handbook [accessed 10 August 2021].

Bowling, A. (2014) *Research Methods in Health* (4th edn). New York: Open University Press.

Bradshaw, A. and Merriman, C. (2008) 'Nursing competence 10 years on: fit for practice and purpose yet?', *Journal of Clinical Nursing*, 17(10): 1263–9.

Brady, N. and Lewin, L. (2007) 'Evidence-based nursing: bridging the gap between research and practice', *Journal of Pediatric Health Care*, 21(1): 53–6.

Butterworth, T., Jackson, C., Brown, L., Orme, M., Fergusson, J. and Hessey, E. (2004) *Developing and sustaining a world class workforce of educators and researchers in health and social care. Phase 2 Strategic Report for StLaR HR Plan Project*. Strategic Learning and Research Advisory Group (StLaR)/ National Health Service University.

Canadian Nurses Association (2009) *Position Statement: Evidence-informed Decision-making and Nursing Practice*. Ottawa.

Carper, B. (1978) 'Fundamental patterns of knowing in nursing', *Advances in Nursing Science*, 1: 13–23.

Carroll, J. and Johnson, E. (1990) *Decision Research: A Field Guide*. Thousand Oaks, CA: Sage.

Centre for Reviews and Dissemination (2009) *Systematic Reviews: CRD's Guidance for Undertaking Reviews in Health Care*. York: Centre for Reviews and Dissemination, University of York. www.york.ac.uk/media/crd/Systematic_Reviews.pdf [accessed 25 August 2021].

Centre for Reviews and Dissemination (2021) *About PROSPERO*. York: Centre for Reviews and Dissemination, University of York. www.crd.york.ac.uk/prospero/ [accessed 17 August 2021].

Chamberlain, P. (2020) 'Knowledge is not everything', *Design for Health*, 4(1): 1–3. https://doi.org/10.1080/24735132.2020.1731203

Chandler, J., Cumpston, M., Thomas, J., Higgins, J.P.T., Deeks, J.J. and Clarke, M.J. (2021) 'Introduction', in J.P.T. Higgins, J. Thomas, J. Chandler, M. Cumpston, T. Li, M.J. Page and V.A. Welch (eds) *Cochrane Handbook for Systematic Reviews of Interventions: version 6.2*. London: Cochrane. https://training.cochrane.org/handbook [accessed 17 August 2021].

Chen, H. (1990) *Theory-Driven Evaluation*. Newbury Park, CA: Sage.

Chen, H. and Rossi, P. (1981) 'The multi-goal theory-driven approach to evaluation: a model linking basic and applied social sciences', in H. Freeman & M. Soloman (eds) *Evaluation Studies Review Annual*, 6. Beverly Hills, CA: Sage pp. 38-54

Chinn, P.L. and Kramer, M.K. (2018) *Knowledge Development in Nursing: Theory and Process* (10th edn). St Louis, MO: Elsevier.

Clark, T. and Holmes, S. (2007) 'Fit for practice? An exploration of the development of newly qualified nurses using focus groups', *International Journal of Nursing Studies.*, 44(1): 1210–20.

Cochrane, A. (1972) *Effectiveness and Efficiency: Random Reflections on the Health Service*. Abingdon: Burgess.

Cochrane, A.L. (1979) '1931–1971: a critical review with particular reference to the medical profession', in *Medicines for the Year 2000*. London: Office of Health Economics. pp. 1-11.

Cochrane Community (2017) *Cochrane's 'logo review' gets an update*. https://community.cochrane.org/news/cochranes-logo-review-gets-update [accessed 17 August 2021].

Cochrane Community (2019) *Living Systematic Reviews*. https://community.cochrane.org/review-production/production-resources/living-systematic-reviews [accessed 25 August 2021].

Colaizzi, P.F. (1978) 'Psychological research as the phenomenologists view it', in R. Valle and M. King (eds) *Existential Phenomenological Alternative for Psychology*. Oxford: Oxford University Press.

Collins, S. and Stockton, C.M. (2018) 'The central role of theory in qualitative research', *International Journal of Qualitative Methods*, 17: 1–10.

Cooke, A., Smith, D. and Booth, A. (2012) 'Beyond PICO: the SPIDER tool for qualitative evidence synthesis', *Qualitative Health Research*, 22(10): 1435–43.

Cormack, D., Gerrish, K. and Lathlean J. (eds) (2015) *The Research Process in Nursing* (3rd edn). Oxford: Wiley-Blackwell.

Council for Training in Evidence-Based Behavioural Practice (2008) *Definition and Competencies for Evidence-Based Behavioural Practice (EBBP)*. https://slidetodoc.com/council-for-training-in-evidence-based-behavioral-practice/ (accessed 27 September 2021).

Craig, J.V. and Stevens, K.R. (2011) 'Evidence-based practice in health care: what is it and why do we need it?', in J.V. Craig and R.L. Smyth (eds) *The Evidence-based Practice Manual for Nurses* (3rd edn). Edinburgh: Churchill Livingstone/Elsevier.

Critical Appraisal Skills Programme (2018) *CASP Qualitative Checklist*. https://casp-uk.b-cdn.net/wp-content/uploads/2018/03/CASP-Qualitative-Checklist-2018_fillable_form.pdf [accessed 25 August 2021].

Crowley, P. (1989) 'Promoting pulmonary maturity', in I. Chalmers, M. Enkin and M.J.N.C. Keirse (eds) *Effective Care in Pregnancy and Childbirth*. Oxford: Oxford University Press. pp. 746–64.

Dale, A.E. (2005) 'Evidence-based practice: compatibility with nursing', *Nursing Standard*, 19(40): 48–53.

Davies, P. (2004) *Is evidence-based government possible?* Jerry Lee Lecture, 2004. Presented at the 4th Annual Campbell Collaboration Colloquium, Washington, DC, National School of Government (UK).

Dawson, D. and Endacott, R. (2011) 'Implementing quality initiatives using bundled approach', *Intensive Critical Care Nursing*, 27: 117–20.

Deeks, J.J., Higgins, J.P.T. and Altman, D.G. (eds) (2021) 'Analysing data and undertaking meta-analyses', in J.P.T. Higgins, J. Thomas, J. Chandler, M. Cumpston, T. Li, M.J. Page and V.A. Welch (eds) *Cochrane Handbook for Systematic Reviews of Interventions: version 6.2*. London: Cochrane. https://training.cochrane.org/handbook [accessed 17 August 2021].

Deming, W.E. (1986) *Out of the Crisis*. Cambridge, MA: MIT Centre for Advanced Engineering Study.

Densen, P. (2011) 'Challenges and opportunities facing medical education', *Transactions of the American Clinical and Climatological Association*, 122: 48–58.

Department of Health (DH) (1989) *Working for Patients*. White Paper. HM Government.

Department of Health (DH) (1997) *The New NHS: Modern and Dependable*. London: HMSO.

Department of Health (DH) (1998) *A First Class Service: Quality in the New NHS*. London: HMSO.

Department of Health (DH) (1999) Health Service Circular – *Making a difference to nursing and midwifery pre-registration education*, HSC 1999/219: 1–18.

Department of Health (DH) (2003) *Building on the Best: Choice, Responsiveness and Equity in the NHS*. London: The Stationery Office.

Department of Health (DH) (2006) *Modernising Nursing Careers: Setting the Direction*. Edinburgh: The Scottish Executive.

Department of Health (DH) (2007) *Report of the High Level Group on Clinical Effectiveness*. London: The Stationery Office.

Department of Health (DH) (2014) *Delivering High Quality, Effective, Compassionate Care: Developing the Right People with the Right Skills and the Right Values. A Mandate from the Government to Health Education England: April 2014 to March 2015*. 1 May 2014. London: The Stationery Office.

Department of Health and Social Care (DHSC) (2021) *The NHS Constitution*. London: The Stationery Office.

Derbyshire, J. (2018) 'Use of scenario planning as a theory-driven evaluation tool', *Futures and Foresight Science*, 1(1): 1-13.

Dewing, J., McCormack, B. and Tichen, A. (2015) *Practice Development Workbook for Nursing, Health and Social Care Teams*. London: Wiley-Blackwell.

DiCenso, A., Cullum, N. and Ciliska, D. (2013) 'Implementing evidence-based nursing: Some misconceptions', in N. Cullum, D. Ciliska, B. Haynes and S. Marks (eds) *Evidence-Based Nursing: An Introduction*. Oxford: Blackwell Publishing.

Dixon-Woods, M., Shaw, R.L., Agarwal, S., et al (2004) 'The problem of appraising qualitative research', *British Medical Journal Quality & Safety*, 13: 223–5.

Dowding, D. and Thompson, C. (2004) 'Using judgement to improve accuracy in decision-making', *Nursing Times*, 100(22): 42–4.

EBSCO (2021) *CINAHL database*. www.ebsco.com/products/research-databases/cinahl-database [accessed 30 July 2021].

EBSCO Connect (2021) *CINAHL subject headings - frequently asked questions*. https://connect.ebsco.com/s/article/CINAHL-Subject-Headings-Frequently-Asked-Questions?language=en_US#:~:text=Total%20Number%20of%20Headings%2015%2C656,References%20for%20the%20Headings%2044%2C410 [accessed 30 July 2021].

Ellis, P. (2010) *Evidence-based Practice in Nursing*. Exeter: Learning Matters.

Eraut, M. (2000) 'Non-formal learning and tacit knowledge in professional work', *British Journal of Educational Psychology*, 70: 113–36.

Evans, D. and Pearson, A (2001) 'Systematic reviews of qualitative research', *Clinical Effectiveness in Nursing*, 5(3): 111–19.

Facione, P. and Gittens, C.A. (2013) *THINK Critically*. London: Pearson.

Fejes, A (2008) 'Governing nursing through reflection: a discourse analysis of reflective practices', *Journal of Advanced Nursing*, 64(3): 243–50.

Fineout-Overholt, E., Melnyk, B.M., Stillwell, S.B. and Williamson, K.M. (2010) 'Evidence-based practice, step by step: critical appraisal of the evidence: part III', *American Journal of Nursing*, 110(11): 43–51.

Finlayson, K. and Dixon, A. (2008) 'Qualitative meta-synthesis: a guide for the novice', *Nurse Researcher*, 15(2): 59–71.

Follett, B. and Paulson-Ellis, M. (2001) *A Review of Appraisal, Disciplinary and Reporting Arrangements for Senior NHS and University Staff with Academic and Clinical Duties.* A Report to the Secretary of State for Education and Skills, by Professor Sir Brian Follett and Michael Paulson-Ellis, September.

Foucault, M. (1979) *The History of Sexuality, Vol.* 1. London: Penguin.

Francis, R. (2013) *Report of the Mid Staffordshire NHS Foundation Trust Public Inquiry.* London: The Stationery Office.

French, P. (1999) 'The development of evidence-based nursing', *Journal of Advanced Nursing*, 29(1): 72–8.

Fulford, K.W.M. (2004) *Whose Values? – A Workbook for Values-Based Practice in Mental Health Care.* London: The Sainsbury Trust for Mental Health.

Fulford, K.W.M. (2008) 'Values-based practice: a new partner to evidence-based practice and a first for psychiatry?', *Mens Sana Monographs*, 6: 10–21.

Fulford, K.W.M. and Stanghellini, G. (2008) 'The third revolution: philosophy into practice in twenty-first century psychiatry', *Dialogues in Philosophy, Mental and Neuro Sciences*, 1: 5–14.

Fulford, K.W.M., Peile, E. and Carroll, H. (2012) *Essentials of Values Based Practice: Clinical Stories Linking Science with People.* Cambridge: Cambridge University Press.

Garside, R. (2014) 'Should we appraise the quality of qualitative research reports for systematic reviews, and if so, how?', *Innovation: The European Journal of Social Science Research*, 27(1): 67–79.

Gawande, A. (2003) *Complications: A Surgeon's Notes on an Imperfect Science.* New York: Picador.

Gerrish, K. (2000) 'Still fumbling along? A comparative study of the newly qualified nurse's perception of the transition from student to qualified nurse', *Journal of Advanced Nursing*, 32(2): 474–80.

Gerrish, K. and Chapman, H. (2017) 'Implementing clinical academic careers in nursing: an exemplar of a large healthcare organisation in the United Kingdom', *Journal of Research in Nursing*, 22(3) 214–25.

Gibbs, G. (1988) *Learning by Doing: A Guide to Teaching and Learning Methods.* Oxford: Further Education Unit, Oxford Polytechnic.

Glaser, B. and Strauss, A. (1967) *The Discovery of Grounded Theory.* Chicago: Aldine.

Glasziou, P. and Haynes, B. (2005) 'The path from research to improved health outcomes', *Evidence-Based Nursing*, 8(2): 36–8.

Glen, S. (2009) 'Nursing education – is it time to go back to the future?', *British Journal of Nursing*, 18(8): 498–502.

Glenton, C., Colvin, C.J., Carlsen, B., Swartz, A., Lewin, S., Noyes, J. and Rashidian, A. (2013) 'Barriers and facilitators to the implementation of lay health worker programmes to improve access to maternal and child health: a qualitative evidence synthesis', *Cochrane Database of Systematic Reviews*, Issue 10. Art. No.: CD010414, https://doi.org/10.1002/14651858.CD010414.pub2 [accessed 19 August 2021].

Goldacre, B. (2011) 'Foreword', in I. Evans, H. Thornton, I. Chalmers and P. Glasziou (eds) *Testing Treatments: Better Research for Better Healthcare* (2nd edn). London: Pinter and Martin.

Goldratt, E. (1999) *Theory of Constraints.* Great Barrington, MA: North River Press.

Gough, D., Oliver, S. and Thomas, J. (2017) *An Introduction to Systematic Reviews* (2nd edn). London: Sage.

Greene, J.C. (2007) *Mixed Methods in Social Inquiry.* San Francisco, CA: John Wiley & Sons

Greenhalgh, T. (1997) 'Getting your bearings (deciding what the paper is about)', *British Medical Journal*, 315: 243–6.

Greenhalgh, T. (2014) *How to Read a Paper: The Basics of Evidence Based Medicine.* (5th edn). New York: John Wiley & Sons

Greenhalgh T. (2017) *How to Implement Evidence-Based Healthcare.* London: Wiley-Blackwell.

Greenhalgh, T. (2019) *How to Read a Paper: The Basics of Evidence-Based Medicine* (6th edn). Oxford: John Wiley & Sons.

Greenway, K., Butt, G. and Walthall, H. (2019) 'What is a theory-practice gap? An exploration of the concept', *Nurse Education in Practice*, 34: 1–6.

Gregory, A., Feder, G., Taket, A. and Williamson, E. (2019) 'Qualitative study to explore the health and well-being impacts on adults providing informal support to female domestic violence survivors', *British Medical Journal Open*, 7: e014511. doi:10.1136/bmjopen-2016-014511.

Grol, R., and Grimshaw, J. (2003) 'From best evidence to best practice: effective implementation of change in patients' care', *Lancet*, 362(9391): 1225-30.

Grol, R., Wensing, M., Eccles, M. and David, D. (eds) (2013) *Improving Patient Care: The Implementation of Change in Health Care* (2nd edn). London: Elsevier.

Guba, E. G., & Lincoln, Y. S. (1989) *Fourth Generation Evaluation*. Newbury Park, CA: Sage Publications, Inc.

Gülmezoglu, A.M., Chandler, J., Shepperd, S. and Pantoja, T. (2013) 'Reviews of qualitative evidence: a new milestone for Cochrane (Editorial)', *Cochrane Database of Systematic Reviews*, 11.

Guyatt, G.H., Oxman, A.D., Schuneman, H.J., Tugwell, P. and Knottnerus, A. (2011) 'GRADE guidelines: a new series of articles in the Journal of Clinical Epidemiology', *Journal of Epidemiology*, 64: 380–2.

Guyatt, G.H., Sackett, D.L. and Cook, D.J. (1994) 'Users' guides to the medical literature. II. How to use an article about therapy or prevention, Part B. What were the results, and will they help me in caring for my patients?', *Evidence-Based Medicine Working Group. JAMA*, 271, 59–63.

Hannes, K. and Lockwood, C. (2011) 'Pragmatism as the philosophical foundation for the Joanna Briggs meta-aggregative approach to qualitative evidence synthesis', *Journal of Advanced Nursing*, 67(7): 1632–42.

Hawkins, P. and Shohet, R. (2012) *Supervision in the Helping Professions*. London: McGraw-Hill Education.

Healthcare Quality Improvement Partnership (2017) *Guide to Managing Ethical Issues in Quality Improvement or Clinical Audit Projects*. London: Healthcare Quality Improvement Partnership Ltd.

Health Education England (HEE) (2014) *Research and Innovation Strategy – Delivering a Flexible Workforce Receptive to Research and Innovation*. London: Department of Health.

Health Education England (HEE) (2015) *Raising the Bar: Shape of Caring: A Review of the Future Education and Training of Registered Nurses and Care Assistants*. Lord Willis, Independent Chair – Shape of Caring review.

Health Education England (HEE) (2021) *Knowledge for Healthcare*. www.hee.nhs.uk/our-work/knowledge-for-healthcare [accessed 26 September 2021]

Health Research Authority (HRA) (2009) *Defining Research*. London: NHS Health Research Authority.

Health Research Authority (HRA) (2017) *UK Policy Framework for Health and Social Care Research*. London: NHS Health Research Authority.

Health Research Authority (HRA) (2018) *UK Policy Framework for Health and Social Care Research*. London: Health Research Authority.

Health Research Authority (HRA) (2020) *UK Policy Framework for Health and Social Care Research*. www.hra.nhs.uk/planning-and-improving-research/policies-standards-legislation/uk-policy-framework-health-social-care-research/

Herbert, R., Jamtvedt, G., Hagen, K.B., Mead, J. and Chambers, I. (2012) *Practical Evidence-Based Physiotherapy* (2nd edn). Edinburgh: Elsevier Butterworth Heinemann.

Higgins, G., Spencer, R. and Kane, R. (2010) 'A systematic review of the experiences and perceptions of the newly qualified nurse in the United Kingdom', *Nurse Education Today*, 30(6): 499–508.

Higgs, J. and Titchen, A. (eds) (2001) *Professional Practice in Health Education and the Creative Arts*. Oxford: Blackwell Science.

Hill, A. and Spittlehouse, C. (2001) *What is Critical Appraisal?* London: Hayward Medical Communications.

Hoffman, K., Dempsey, J., Levett-Jones, T., Noble, D., Hickey, N., Jeong, S., Hunter, S. and Norton, C. (2010) 'The design and implementation of an Interactive Computerised Decision Support Framework (ICDSF) as a strategy to improve nursing students' clinical reasoning skills', *Nurse Education Today*, 31(6): 587–94.

Huntington, A.D. and Gilmour, J.A. (2001) 'Rethinking representations, rewriting nursing texts: possibilities through feminism and Foucauldian thought', *Journal of Advanced Nursing*, 35(6): 902–8.

Iles, V. and Sutherland, K. (2001) *Managing Change in the NHS. Organisational Change: A Review for Health Care Managers, Professionals and Researchers*. London: National Co-ordinating Centre for NHS Service Delivery and Organisation.

Ingersoll, G.L. (2000) 'Evidence-based nursing: what it is and what it isn't', *Nursing Outlook*, 48: 151–2.

Institute for Healthcare Improvement (2012) *What is a Bundle?* www.ihi.org/knowledge/Pages/ImprovementStories/WhatIsaBundle.aspx

Jarvis, I.L. (1972) *Victims of Groupthink: A Psychological Study of Foreign-policy Decisions and Fiascos*. Boston: Houghton Mifflin.

Jasper, M. (1996) 'The first year as a staff nurse: the experiences of a first cohort of Project 2000 nurses in a demonstration district', *Journal of Advanced Nursing*, 24: 779–90.

Jennings, E.T. and Hall, J.L. (2011) 'Evidence-based practice and the use of information in state agency decision making', *Journal of Public Administration Research and Theory*, 22(2): 245–66.

Jungermann, H. and Fischer, K. (2005) 'Using expertise and experience for giving and taking advice', in T. Betsch and S. Haberstroh (eds) *The Routines of Decision Making*. Mahwah, NJ: Lawrence Erlbaum Associates.

Justice, L.M. (2010) 'When craft and science collide: improving therapeutic practices through evidence-based innovations', *International Journal of Speech-Language Pathology*, 12(2): 79–86.

Kaplan, S. A. and Garrett, K. E. (2005) 'The use of logic models by community-based initiatives', *Evaluation and Programme Planning*, 28: 167-72.

Kazi, M. A. F., Blom, B., Moren, S, Perdal, A. L. and Rostila, I. (2002) 'Realistic evaluation for practice in Sweden, Finland and Britain', *Journal of Social Work Research and Evaluation*, 3(2): 171–86.

Kerlinger, F.N. (1999) *Foundations of Behavioural Research* (4th edn). New York: Holt, Rinehart & Winston.

Khan, K., Kunz, R., Kleijnen, J. and Antes, G. (2011) *Systematic Reviews to Support Evidence-Based Medicine: How to Review and Apply Findings of Healthcare Research* (2nd edn). Boca Raton, FL: CRC Press.

King's Fund (2000) *Getting Better with Evidence. Experiences of Putting Evidence into Practice*. London: King's Fund Publishing.

King's Fund (2015) *Staff Engagement. Six Building Blocks for Harnessing the Creativity and Enthusiasm of NHS Staff*. London: King's Fund.

King's Fund (2016) Michael West, Head of Thought Leadership. *If it's about NHS Culture, it's about Leadership*. London: The King's Fund.

King's Fund (2019) *The NHS long-term plan explained*. www.kingsfund.org.uk/publications/nhs-long-term-plan-explained [accessed 26 September 2021].

Kinsella, E. (2010) 'The art of reflective practice in health and social care: reflections on the legacy of Donald Schon', *Reflective Practice: International and Multidisciplinary Perspectives*, 11(4): 565–75.

Kitson, A. (1994) *Clinical Nursing Practice Development and Research Activity in the Oxford Region*. Oxford: National Institute for Nursing/Centre for Practice Development and Research.

Kitson, A. (2002) 'Recognising relationships: reflections on evidence-based practice', *Nursing Inquiry*, 9(3): 179–86.

Kolb, D.A. (2015) *Experiential Learning: Experience as the Source of Learning and Development* (2nd edn). Upper Saddle River: Pearson Education Inc.

Kozlowski, D., Hutchinson, M., Hurley, J., Rowley, J., and Sutherland, J. (2017) 'The role of emotion in clinical decision making: an integrative literature review', *British Medical Council of Medical Education*, 17(1): 255.

Kristensen, N., Nymann, C. and Konradsen, H. (2016) 'Implementing research results in clinical practice – the experiences of healthcare professionals', *British Medical Council Health Research*, 16: 48.

Kuhn, T. (1970) *The Structure of Scientific Revolution* (2nd edn). Chicago: University of Chicago Press.

Lachal, J., Revah-Levy, A., Orri, M. and Moro, M.R. (2017) 'Metasynthesis: an original method to synthesize qualitative literature in psychiatry', *Frontiers in Psychiatry*, 8: 269.

Lamb, B. and Sevdalis, N. (2011) 'How do nurses make decisions?', *International Journal of Nursing Studies*, 48: 281–4.

Lansisalmi, H., Kivimaki, M., Aalto, P. and Ruoranen, R. (2006) 'Innovation in healthcare: a systematic review of recent research', *Nursing Science Quarterly*, 19: 66-72.

Lasater, K. (2007) 'Clinical judgement development: using simulation to create an assessment rubric', *Journal of Nurse Education*, 46(11): 496–503.

Lave, J. and Wenger, E. (1991) *Situated Learning: Legitimate Peripheral Participation*. Cambridge: University of Cambridge Press.

Lehane, E., Leahy-Warren, P., O'Riordan, C., Savage, E., Drennan, J., O'Tuathaigh, C., O'Connor, M., Corrigan, M., Burke, F., Hayes, M., Lynch, H., Sahm, L., Heffernan, E., O'Keeffe, E., Blake, C., Horgan, F. and Hegarty, J. (2018) 'Evidence-based practice education for healthcare professions: an expert view', *British Medical Journal of Evidence Based Medicine*, 24(3): 103–8.

Leininger, M.M. (1985) *Qualitative Research Methods in Nursing*. Orlando, FL: Grune and Stratton.

Levett-Jones, T., Hoffman, K., Dempsey, J., Jeoong, S.Y., Noble, D., Norton, C.A., Roche, J. and Hickey, N. (2010) 'The "five rights" of clinical reasoning: an educational model to enhance nursing students' ability to identify and manage clinically "at risk" patients', *Nurse Education Today*, 30: 515–20.

Lewin, K. (1951) *Field Theory in Social Sciences*. New York: Harper Row.

Lindsay, B. (2007) *Understanding Research and Evidence-based Practice*. Exeter: Reflect Press.

Lizarondo, L., Stern, C., Carrier, J., Godfrey, C., Rieger, K., Salmond, S., Apostolo, J., Kirkpatrick, P. and Loveday, H. (2020) 'Mixed methods systematic reviews', in E. Aromataris and Z. Munn (eds) *JBI Manual for Evidence Synthesis*. Adelaide: JBI.

LoBiondo-Wood, G. and Haber, J. (2017) *Nursing Research: Methods and Critical Appraisal for Evidence-based Practice*. St. Louis, MO: Mosby Elsevier.

Lockwood, C., Munn, Z. and Porritt, K. (2015) 'Qualitative research synthesis', *International Journal of Evidence-Based Healthcare*, 13(3): 179–87.

Lockwood, C., Porrit, K., Munn, Z., Rittenmeyer, L., Salmond, S., Bjerrum, M., Loveday, H., Carrier, J. and Stannard, D. (2020) 'Systematic reviews of qualitative evidence', in E. Aromataris and Z. Munn (eds) *JBI Manual for Evidence Synthesis*. Adelaide: JBI.

Long, A.F., Godfrey, M., Randall, T., Brettle, A.J. and Grant, M.J. (2002) *Developing Evidence Based Social Care Policy and Practice. Part 3: Feasibility of Undertaking Systematic Reviews in Social Care*. Leeds: Nuffield Institute for Health.

Maben, J. and Macleod-Clark, J. (1998) 'Making the transition from student to staff nurse', *Nursing Times*, 92(44): 28–31.

Macdonald, H., Loder, E. and Abbasi, K. (2020) 'Living systematic reviews at The BMJ', *BMJ*, 370: m2925. https://doi: 10.1136/bmj.m2925

MacGuire, J.M. (1990) 'Putting nursing research findings into practice: research utilization as an aspect of the management of change', *Journal of Advanced Nursing*, 15, 614–20.

Maguire, B.J. and Guérin, P.J. (2020) 'A living systematic review protocol for COVID-19 clinical trial registrations', *Wellcome Open Research*, 5(60). https://doi.org/10.12688/wellcomeopenres.15821.1

Maher, L. and Panny, J. (2005) 'Service improvement', in E. Peck (ed.) *Organisational Development in Healthcare: Approaches, Innovations and Achievement*. Oxford: Radcliffe Publishing.

Manicas, P.T. & Secord, P. F. (1983) 'Implication for psychology of the new philosophy of science', *American Psychologist*, 38(4): 399–413.

Manley, K., Hardy, S., Titchen, A., Garbett, R. and McCormack, B. (2005) *Changing Patients' Worlds through Nursing Expertise*. London: Royal College of Nursing.

Manley, K., McCormack, B., Wilson, V. and Thoms, D. (2008) 'The future contribution of practice development in a changing healthcare context', in K. Manley, B. McCormack and V. Wilson (eds) *International Practice Development in Nursing and Healthcare*. Oxford: Blackwell.

Mantzoukas, S. (2008) 'The research evidence published in high impact nursing journals between 2000 and 2006: a quantitative content analysis', *International Journal of Nursing Studies*, 46: 479–89.

Martin-Ferreres, M.L., De Juan Pardo, M.Á., Bardallo Porras, D. and Medina Moya, J.L. (2019) 'An ethnographic study of human dignity in nursing practice', *Nursing Outlook*, 67(4): 393–403.

Mason, T. and Mason-Whitehead, E. (2011) *Foundations of Nursing Theory* (2nd edn). Maidenhead: Open University Press.

Mavergames, C. and Elliott, J. (n.d.) 'Living systematic reviews: towards real-time evidence for healthcare decision-making', *BMJ Best Practice*. https://bestpractice.bmj.com/info/toolkit/discuss-ebm/living-systematic-reviews-towards-real-time-evidence-for-health-care-decision-making/ [accessed 25 August 2021].

McGonagle, I., Jackson, C. and Kane, R. (2015) 'The ten essential shared capabilities: reflections on education in values based practice: a qualitative study', *Nurse Education Today*, 35(2): e24–e28.

McLean, C. (2011) 'Change and transition: navigating the journey', *British Journal of School Nursing*, 6(3): 141–5.

McPhail, G. (1997) 'Management of change: an essential skill for nursing in the 1990s', *Journal of Nursing Management*, 5: 199–205.

McSherry, R., Artley, A. and Holland, J. (2006) 'Research awareness: an important factor for evidence-based practice?', *Worldviews on Evidence-Based Nursing*, 3: 113–17.

Melnyk, B.M. and Fineout-Overholt, E. (2018) *Evidence-based Practice in Nursing and Healthcare: A Guide to Best Practice* (4th edn). Philadelphia: Wolters Kluwer.

Menon, S., Karl, J., & Wignaraja, K. (2009) *Handbook on Planning, Monitoring and Evaluating for Development Results*. New York: United Nations Development Programme.

Metz, A.J.R., Blasé, K. and Bowie, L. (2007) 'Implementing evidence-based practices: six drivers of success. Brief research-to-results', *Child Trends*, October.

Miller, S.A. and Forrest, J.J. (2001) 'Enhancing your practice decision making: PICO, learning how to ask good questions', *Journal of Evidence-Based Dental Practice*, 1: 136–41.

Miyata, H. and Kai, I. (2009) 'Reconsidering evaluation criteria for scientific adequacy in health care research: an integrative framework of quantitative and qualitative criteria', *International Journal of Qualitative Methods*, 8(1): 64–75.

Mohajan, H.K. (2018) 'Qualitative research methodology in social sciences and related subjects', *Journal of Economic Development, Environment and People*, 7(1): 23–48.

Mohanna K. (2017) 'Values based practice: a framework for thinking with', *Education in Primary Care*, 28(4): 192–6. doi: 10.1080/14739879.2017.1313689

Moher, D., Liberati, A., Tetzlaff, J., Altman, D.G. and The PRISMA Group (2009) 'Preferred reporting items for systematic reviews and meta-analyses: the PRISMA statement', *PLoS Medicine*, 6(7): e1000097.

Moher, D., Shamseer, L., Clarke, M., Ghersi, D., Liberati, A., Petticrew, P.S., Stewart, L.A. and PRISMA-P Group (2015) 'Preferred reporting items for systematic review and meta-analysis protocols (PRISMA-P) 2015 statement', *Systematic Reviews*, 4(1). https://doi.org/10.1186/2046-4053-4-1

Monaghan, T. (2015) 'A critical analysis of the literature and theoretical perspectives on theory–practice gap amongst newly qualified nurses within the United Kingdom', *Nurse Education Today*, 35(8): 1–7.

Moola, S., Munn, Z., Sears, K., Sfetcu, R., Currie, M., Lisy, K., Tufanaru, C., Qureshi, R., Mattis, P. and Mu, P. (2015) 'Conducting systematic reviews of association (etiology): the Joanna Briggs Institute's approach', *International Journal of Evidence-Based Healthcare*, 13(3): 163–9.

Moorley, C. and Cathala, X. (2019) 'How to appraise qualitative research', *Evidence-Based Nursing*, 22: 10–13.

Morse, J.M. (1991) 'Approaches to qualitative-quantitative methodological triangulation', *Nursing Research*, 40: 120–3.

Moule, P., Aveyard, H. and Goodman, M. (2016) *Nursing Research: An Introduction* (3rd edn). London: Sage.

Muir Gray, J.A. (1997) *Evidence-based Healthcare: How to Make Health Policy and Management Decisions*. London: Churchill Livingstone.

Mullhall, P.L. (1993) 'Unknowing: towards another pattern of knowing', *Nursing Outlook*, 41: 125–8.

Muntean, W. (2012) 'Nursing clinical decision-making: a literature review'. www.semanticscholar.org/paper/Nursing-Clinical-Decision-Making-%3A-A-Literature-Muntean/ba14b0d8ef4006ebdd03b73bd62355001f436ee2#citing-papers [accessed 28 September 2021].

Nairn, S. (2012) 'A critical realists' approach to knowledge: implications for evidence-based practice in and beyond nursing', *Nursing Inquiry*, 19(1): 6–17.

National Institute for Health and Care Excellence (NICE) (2002) *Principles for Best Practice in Clinical Audit*. Oxon: Radcliffe Medical Press Ltd.

National Institute for Health and Care Excellence (NICE) (2014) *Developing NICE Guidelines: The Manual*. www.nice.org.uk/media/default/about/what-we-do/our-programmes/developing-nice-guidelines-the-manual.pdf [accessed 17 January 2022].

National Institute for Health and Care Excellence (NICE) (2020) *Developing NICE Guidelines: The Manual (PMG20)*. www.nice.org.uk/process/pmg20/resources/developing-nice-guidelines-the-manual-pdf-72286708700869 [accessed 17 August 2021].

National Institute for Health Research (2016) *Building a Research Career: A Guide for Aspiring Clinical Academics and their Managers*. London: NHS National Institute for Health Research.

National Institute for Health Research (2018) *Patient and Public Involvement in Health and Social Care Research*. London: NHS National Institute for Health Research.

NHS (2019) 'Patient experience in adult NHS services: improving the experience of care for people using adult NHS services', Clinical guideline [CG138] www.nice.org.uk/guidance/cg138/chapter/1-guidance [accessed 25 September 2021].

NHS (2021) *NHS Long Term Plan*. www.longtermplan.nhs.uk/ [accessed 26 September 2021].

NHS (2021) *The NHS Constitution: All You Need to Know About How the NHS Constitution Affects You As A Provider or Commissioner of NHS Care*. London: DH Publications.

NHS Digital (2021) 'NHS pathways'. https://digital.nhs.uk/services/nhs-pathways [accessed 5 August 2021].

NHS Education for Scotland (2010) *National Guidance for Clinical Academic Research Careers for Nursing, Midwifery and Allied Health Professions in Scotland*. Edinburgh: NHS Education for Scotland.

NHS Education for Scotland (2021) *Core Skills of Clinical Decision Making*. www.effectivepractitioner.nes.scot.nhs.uk/clinical-practice/core-skills-of-decision-making.aspx [accessed 05.01.22].

NHS England (2016) *Leading Change, Adding Value*. www.england.nhs.uk/wp-content/uploads/2016/05/nursing-framework.pdf

NHS England (2017) *Building Greater Insight Through Qualitative Research. 05 / Bite-Size Guide to Patient Insight*. Publications gateway reference: 06757. London: NHS England.

NHS England and NHS Improvement (2019) *Building Collaborative Teams*. www.england.nhs.uk/improvement-hub/publication/building-collaborative-teams/ [accessed 26 September 2021].

NHS England and NHS Improvement (2019) *Plan, Do, Study, Act (PDSA) Cycles and the Model for Improvement.* London: NHS England and NHS Improvement.

NHS England and NHS Improvement (2021) *Online Library of Quality, Service Improvement and Redesign Tools: Plan, Do, Study, Act (PDSA) cycles and the model for improvement.* London: NHS England and NHS Improvement.

NHS Executive (1996) *Promoting Clinical Effectiveness: A Framework for Action in and through the NHS.* Leeds: NHS Executive.

NHS Institute for Innovation and Improvement (2005) *Improvement Leaders' Guide: Managing the Human Dimensions of Change, Personal and Organisational Development.* www.institute.nhs.uk/ improvementleadersguides

NHS Leadership Academy (2016) *Developing People – Improving Care: A National Framework for Action on Improvement and Leadership Development in NHS-funded Services.* London: NHS Leadership Academy.

NHS Scottish Executive (2006) *National Quality Standards for Substance Misuse Services.* Edinburgh: Scottish Executive.

Nibbelink, C. W., and Brewer, B. B. (2018) 'Decision-making in nursing practice: an integrative literature review', *Journal of Clinical Nursing,* 27(5-6): 917–28.

Nickols, F. (2016) 'Six factors affecting performance alignment', *Performance Improvement* 55(3): 6–9.

Nielsen, A., Stragnell, M.S. and Jester, P. (2007) 'Guide for reflection using the Clinical Judgement Model', *Journal of Nursing Education,* 46(11): 513–16.

Nieswiadomy, R.M. and Bailey C. (2017) *Foundations of Nursing Research* (7th edn). Cranbury, NJ: Pearson Education.

Noblit, G. and Hare, R.D. (1988) *Meta-ethnography: Synthesizing Qualitative Studies.* Newbury Park, CA: Sage.

Norcross J.C. and Wampold, B.E. (2018) 'A new therapy for each patient: evidence-based relationships and responsiveness', *Journal of Clinical Psychology.* 74(11): 1889–906.

Noyes, J., Booth, A., Cargo, M., Flemming, K., Harden, A., Harris, J., Garside, R., Hannes, K., Pantoja, T. and Thomas, J. (2021) 'Qualitative evidence', in J.P.T. Higgins, J. Thomas, J. Chandler, M. Cumpston, T. Li, M.J. Page and V.A. Welch (eds) *Cochrane Handbook for Systematic Reviews of Interventions: version 6.2.* London: Cochrane. https://training.cochrane.org/handbook [accessed 25 August 2021].

Nursing and Midwifery Council (NMC) (2018a) *Future Nurse: Standards of Proficiency for Registered Nurses.* London: NMC.

Nursing and Midwifery Council (NMC) (2018b) *The Code: Professional Standards of Practice and Behaviour for Nurses, Midwives and Nursing Associates.* London: NMC.

Nursing and Midwifery Council (NMC) (2019) *Revalidation: How to Revalidate with the NMC. Requirements for Renewing your Registration.* London: NMC.

Omachonu, V.K. and Einspruch, N.G. (2010) 'Innovation in health care delivery systems: a conceptual framework', *The Public Sector Innovation Journal,* 51(1): 1–20.

Ormston, R., Spencer, L., Barnard, K. and Snape, D. (2018) 'The foundations of qualitative research', in J. Ritchie, J. Lewis, C. McNaughton Nicholls and R. Ormston (eds) *Qualitative Research Practice: A Guide for Social Science Students and Researchers* (2nd edn). London: Sage. pp. 1–23.

Oxford English Dictionary (2021) *Oxford English Dictionary Online.* www.oed.com/ [accessed 10 August 2021].

Page, M.J., McKenzie, J.E., Bossuyt, P.M., Boutron, I., Hoffmann, T.C., Mulrow, C.D., Shamseer, L., Tetzlaff, J.M., Akl, E.A., Brennan, S.E., Chou, R., Glanville, J., Grimshaw, J.M., Hróbjartsson, A., Lalu, M.M., Li, T., Loder, E.W., Mayo-Wilson, E. McDonald, S., McGuinness, L.A., Stewart, L.A., Thomas, J., Tricco, A.C., Welch, V.A., Whiting, P. and Moher, D. (2021) 'The PRISMA 2020 statement: an updated guideline for reporting systematic reviews', *BMJ,* 372: n71. http://dx.doi. org/10.1136/bmj.n71

Page, S. and Hammer, S. (2002) 'Practice development – time to realize the potential', *Practice Development in Health Care*, 1(1): 2–17.

Pape, T.M. (2003) 'Evidence-based nursing practice: to infinity and beyond', *The Journal of Continuing Education in Nursing*, 34(4): 154–61.

Parahoo, K. (2014) *Nursing Research: Principles, Process and Issues* (3rd edn). Basingstoke: Palgrave Macmillan.

Pawson, R. (2002) 'Evidence-based policy: in search of a method', *Evaluation*, 8(2): 157–81.

Pawson, R. and Tilley, N. (1997) *Realistic Evaluation*. Thousand Oaks, CA: Sage.

Pearson, A. (2005) 'A broader view of evidence', *International Journal of Nursing Practice*, 11(3): 93–4.

Pearson, A., Field, J. and Jordan, Z. (2007) *Evidence-based Clinical Practice in Nursing and Health Care: Assimilating Research, Experience and Expertise*. Oxford: Blackwell Publishing.

Pearson, A., White, H., Bath-Hextall, F., Salmond, S., Apostolo, J. and Kirkpatrick, P. (2015) 'A mixed-methods approach to systematic reviews', *International Journal of Evidence-Based Healthcare*, 13(3): 121–31.

Peile, E. (2004) 'Reflections from medical practice: balancing evidence-based practice with practice-based evidence', in G. Thomas and R. Pring (eds) *Evidence-Based Practice in Education*. Maidenhead: Open University Press.

Penny, J. (2003) 'Discipline of improvement in health and social care', in NHS Institute for Innovation and Improvement (2005) *Improvement Leaders Guide: Improvement Knowledge and Skills*. London: NHS Institute for Innovation and Improvement.

Petrova, M., Dale, J. and Fulford, K.W.M. (2006) 'Values-based practice in primary care: easing the tensions between individual values, ethical principles and best evidence', *British Journal of General Practice*, 56(530): 703–9.

Petticrew, M. and Roberts, H. (2003) 'Evidence, hierarchies and typologies: horses for courses', *Journal of Epidemiology and Community Health*, 57: 527–9.

Petticrew, M. and Roberts, H. (2006) *Systematic Reviews in the Social Sciences: A Practical Guide*. Malden, MA: Blackwell Publishing.

Polit, D.F. and Beck, C.T. (2018) *Essentials of Nursing Research: Appraising Evidence for Nursing Practice* (9th international edn). Philadelphia: Wolters Kluwer.

Polit, D.F. and Beck, C.T. (2020) *Essentials of Nursing Research: Appraising Evidence for Nursing Practice* (10th edn). Philadelphia: Wolters Kluwer.

Porter, S. and O'Halloran, P. (2012) 'The use and limitation of realistic evaluation as a tool for evidence-based practice: a critical realist perspective', *Nursing Inquiry*, 19(1): 18–28.

Price, R. (2009) 'Diploma to degree 1976–1993', *Radiography*, 15(Suppl 1): e67–e71.

PRISMA (2021a) *Preferred Reporting Items for Systematic Reviews and Meta-Analyses (PRISMA)*. www.prisma-statement.org/ [accessed 17 August 2021].

PRISMA (2021b) 'PRISMA endorsers list'. www.prisma-statement.org/Endorsement/PRISMAEndorsers [accessed 17 August 2021].

Reed, M. S., Vella, S., Challies E., de Vente, J., Frewer, L., Hohenwallner-Ries, D., et al. (2017) 'A theory of participation: what makes stakeholder and public engagement in environmental management work?' *Restoration Ecology*, 26 (S1): S7–S17.

Rethlefsen, M.L., Kirtley, S., Waffenschmidt, S., Ayala, A.P., Moher, D., Page, M.J., Koffel, J.B. and PRISMA-S Group (2021) 'PRISMA-S: an extension to the PRISMA Statement for Reporting Literature Searches in Systematic Reviews', *Systematic Reviews*, 10: 39. https://doi.org/10.1186/s13643-020-01542-z

Richardson, W.S., Wilson, M.C., Nishikawa, J. and Hayward, R.S. (1995) 'The well-built clinical question: a key to evidence-based decisions', *ACP Journal Club*, 123(2): A12–3.

Rooddehghan, Z., ParsaYekta, Z. and Nasrabadi, A.N. (2019) 'Equity in nursing care: a grounded theory study', *Nursing Ethics*, 26(2): 598–610.

Rossi, P. H. and Freeman, H. E. (1985) *Evaluation: A Systematic Approach*. Beverly-Hills, CA: Sage Publications.

Rossi, P., Lipsey, M.W. and Freeman, H. (2004) *Evaluation: A Systematic Approach* (7th edn). Thousand Oaks, CA: Sage.

Royal College of General Practitioners (2021) 'Innovation'. www.rcgp.org.uk/clinical-and-research/our-programmes/innovation.aspx [accessed 26 September 2021].

Royal College of Nursing (2007) *Helping Students Get the Best from their Clinical Placements*. London: RCN.

Royal College of Physicians (2019) *Personalizing Healthcare: The Role of Shared Decision Making and Support for Self-Management, RCP Position Statement*. London: Royal College of Physicians.

Rycroft-Malone, J. (2004) 'The PARIHS Framework – a framework for guiding the implementation of evidence-based practice', *Journal of Nursing Care Quality*, 19(4): 297–304.

Rycroft-Malone, J., Seers, K., Titchen, A., Harvey, G., Kitson, A. and McCormack, B. (2004) 'What counts as evidence in evidence-based practice?', *Journal of Advanced Nursing*, 47(1): 81–90.

Sackett, D.L., Rosenberg, W.M.C., Grey, J.A.M., Haynes, R.B. and Richardson, W.S. (1996) 'Evidence based medicine: what it is and what it isn't. It's about integrating individual clinical expertise and the best external evidence', *British Medical Journal*, 312(7023): 71–2.

Sackett, D.L., Straus, S.E., Scott-Richardson, W., Rosenberg, W.M.C., Grey, J.A.M. and Haynes, R.B. (2000) *Evidence-based Medicine: How to Practice and Teach EBM*. London: Churchill Livingstone.

Salama, R. (2010) *Monitoring and Evaluation of Health Services*. Online Presentation. https://sites.pitt.edu/~super4/37011-38001/37851.ppt [accessed 24 September 2021].

Sandelowski, M. and Barroso, J. (2007) *Handbook for Synthesizing Qualitative Research*. New York: Springer.

Sanderlin, B.W. and Abdul Rahhim, N. (2007) 'Evidence-based medicine, Part 6: an introduction to critical appraisal of clinical practice guidelines', *Journal of the American Osteopathic Association*, 107(8): 321–4.

Sandstrom, B., Borglin, G., Nilsson, R., et al. (2015) 'Promoting the implementation of evidence-based practice: a literature review focusing on the role of nursing leadership', *Worldviews on Evidence-Based Nursing*, 8(4): 212–23.

Sayer, R. A. (2000) *Realism and Social Science*. London: Sage.

Scambler, G. (2018) *Basic Critical Realism and Health*. London: Routledge.

Schön, D.A. (1990) *Educating the Reflective Practitioner: Toward a New Design for Teaching and Learning in the Professions*. The Jossey-Bass Higher Education series. San Francisco, CA: Jossey-Bass.

Schön, D.A. (1994) *The Reflective Practitioner: How Professionals Think in Action*. New York: Basic Books.

Schulz, K.F., Altman, D.G. and Moher, D., for the CONSORT Group (2010) 'CONSORT 2010 Statement: Updated guidelines for reporting parallel group randomised trials', *BMJ*, 340: c332.

Scott, K. and McSherry, R. (2008) 'Evidence-based nursing: clarifying the concepts in nursing practice', *Journal of Clinical Nursing*, 18: 1085–95.

Shaban, R.Z., Considine, J., Fry, M. and Curtis, K. (2017) 'Case study and case-based research in emergency nursing and care: theoretical foundations and practical application in paramedic pre-hospital clinical judgement and decision-making of patients with mental illness', *Australian Emergency Nursing Journal*, 20: 17–24.

Shadish, W. R., Cook, T. D. and Campbell, D. T. (2002) *Experimental and Quasi-Experimental Designs for Generalized Causal Inference*. Boston: Houghton Mifflin.

Sibson, R. and Riebe, L. (2016) *Developing professional identity through self-reflection using an ePortfolio app*. In ePortfolios Australia Forum 2016: Connecting learning to the future. Queensland, Australia: Queensland University of Technology.

Smith R. (1992) 'Audit and research'. *BMJ*; 305: 905-6.

Social Care Institute for Excellence (SCIE) (2019) *Using results to continuously improve integrated care.* SCIE online: www.scie.org.uk/integrated-care/better-care/guides/measure-impact/improve [accessed 24 September 2021].

Soilemezi, D. and Lincenviciute, S. (2018) 'Synthesizing qualitative research: reflections and lessons learnt by two new reviewers', *International Journal of Qualitative Methods*, 17: 1–14.

Spencer, L., Ritchie, J., Lewis, J. and Dillon, L. (2003) *Quality in Qualitative Evaluation: A Framework for Assessing Research Evidence.* London: National Centre for Social Research.

Standing, M. (2017) *Clinical Judgement and Decision Making in Nursing* (3rd edn). Transforming Nursing Practice series. London: Sage.

Stenfors, T., Kajamaa, A. and Bennett, D. (2020) 'How to … assess the quality of qualitative research', *The Clinical Teacher*, 17: 596–9.

Sterne, J.A.C., Savović, J., Page, M.J., Elbers, R.G., Blencowe, N.S., Boutron, I., Cates, C.J., Cheng, H-Y., Corbett, M.S., Eldridge, S.M., Hernán, M.A., Hopewell, S., Hróbjartsson, A., Junqueira, D.R., Jüni, P., Kirkham, J.J., Lasserson, T., Li, T., McAleenan, A., Reeves, B.C., Shepperd, S., Shrier, I., Stewart, L.A., Tilling, K., White, I.R., Whiting, P.F. and Higgins, J.P.T. (2019) 'RoB 2: a revised tool for assessing risk of bias in randomised trials', *BMJ*, 366: l4898. https://doi.org/10.1136/bmj.l4898

Stevens, K.R. (2013) 'The impact of evidence-based practice in nursing and the next big ideas', *Online Journal of Issues in Nursing*, 18(2): 4.

Stillwell, S.B., Fineout-Overholt, E., Melnyk, B.M. and Williamson, K.M. (2010) 'Asking the clinical question: a key step in evidence-based practice', *American Journal of Nursing*, 110(3): 58–61.

Straus, S.E., Glasziou, P., Richardson, W.S. and Haynes, R.B. (2019) *Evidence-based Medicine: How to Practice and Teach EBM* (5th edn). Edinburgh: Churchill Livingstone.

Strauss, A. and Corbin, J.M. (1990) *Basics of Qualitative Research: Grounded Theory, Procedures and Techniques.* Thousand Oaks, CA: Sage.

Streubert, H.J. and Carpenter, D.R. (2010) *Qualitative Research in Nursing: Advancing the Humanistic Imperative* (5th edn). Philadelphia: Lippincott Williams and Wilkins.

Stricktland K (2017) 'Developing an infrastructure to support clinical academic careers', *British Journal of Nursing*, 26(22): 1249-52.

Sutton, A., Clowes, M., Preston, L. and Booth, A. (2019) 'Meeting the review family: exploring review types and associated information retrieval requirements', *Health Information and Libraries Journal*, 36(3): 202–22.

Sutton, R.T., Pincock, D., Baumgart, D.C., Sadowski, D.C., Fedorak, R.N. and Kroeker, K.I. (2020) 'An overview of clinical decision support systems: benefits, risks, and strategies for success', *NPJ Digital Medicine*, 3:17.

Tanner, C.A. (2006) 'Thinking like a nurse: a research-based model of clinical judgement in nursing', *Journal of Nurse Education*, 45(6): 204–11.

Taylor, B. (2000) *Reflective Practice: A Guide for Nurses and Midwives.* London: Allen & Unwin; Melbourne: Open University Press.

Thomas, G. (2004) 'Introduction: evidence and practice', in G. Thomas and R. Pring (eds) *Evidence-based Practice in Education: Conducting Educational Research.* Maidenhead: Open University Press.

Thompson, C. (2003) 'Clinical experience as evidence in evidence-based practice', *Journal of Advanced Nursing*, 43(3): 230–7.

Thompson, C., Cullum, N. and McCaughan, D. (2004) 'Nurse, information use and clinical decision making – real world potential for evidence-based decisions in nursing', *Evidence Based Nursing*, 7: 68–72.

Timmins, F., McCabe, C. and McSherry, R. (2012) 'Research awareness: managerial challenges for nurses in the Republic of Ireland', *Journal of Nursing Management*, 20: 224–35.

Tong, A., Flemming, K., McInnes, E., Oliver, S. and Craig, J. (2012) 'Enhancing transparency in reporting the synthesis of qualitative research: ENTREQ', *BMC Medical Research Methodology*, 12: 181. https://doi.org/10.1186/1471-2288-12-181

Tricco, A.C., Antony, J., Zarin, W., Strifler, L., Ghassemi, M., Ivory, J., Perrier, L., Hutton, B., Moher, D. and Straus, S.E. (2015) 'A scoping review of rapid review methods', *BMC Medicine*, 13: 224. https://doi.org/10.1186/s12916-015-0465-6.

Twycross, A. and Shorten, A. (2014) 'Service evaluation, audit and research: what is the difference?' *Evidence Based Nursing*, 17(3): 65–6.

United Kingdom Central Council for Nursing, Midwifery and Health Visiting (UKCC) (1986) *Project 2000: A New Preparation for Practice, United Kingdom Central Council for Nursing, Midwifery and Health Visiting*. London: UKCC.

United Kingdom Central Council for Nursing, Midwifery and Health Visiting (UKCC) (1999) *Fitness for Practice: The UKCC Commission for Nursing and Midwifery Education, United Kingdom Central Council for Nursing, Midwifery and Health Visiting*. London: UKCC.

United Kingdom Clinical Research Collaboration Subcommittee for Nurses in Clinical Research (UKCRC) (Workforce) (2007) *Developing the Best Research Professionals. Qualified Graduate Nurses: Recommendations for Preparing and Supporting Clinical Academic Nurses of the Future. The 'Finch' Report*. London: UKCRC.

University of Waterloo (2015) 'Group decision making', Centre for Teaching Excellence. https://uwaterloo.ca/centre-for-teaching-excellence/teaching-resources/teaching-tips/developing-assignments/group-work/group-decision-making [accessed 28 September 2021].

US National Library of Medicine (2020) 'Citations added to MEDLINE® by fiscal year'. www.nlm.nih.gov/bsd/stats/cit_added.html [accessed 29 July 2021].

US National Library of Medicine (2021) 'MEDLINE: overview'. www.nlm.nih.gov/medline/medline_overview.html [accessed 29 July 2021].

Van Graan, A.C. and Williams, M.J.S. (2017) 'A conceptual framework to facilitate clinical judgement in nursing: a methodological perspective', *Health Gesondheid*, 22: 275–90.

Wade, D. (2005) 'Ethics, audit, and research: all shades of grey', *BMJ*, 330: 468.

Weiss, C. (1995) 'Nothing as practical as good theory: Exploring theory-based evaluation for comprehensive community initiatives for children and families', in J. P. Connell, A. C. Kubisch, L. B. Schorr and C. H. Weiss (eds) *New Approaches to Evaluating Community Initiatives: Vol. 1, Concepts, Methods, and Contexts*. Washington, DC: The Aspen Institute. pp 65–92.

Weiss, C. H. (2000) 'Theory-based evaluation: Theories of change for poverty reduction programs', in O. Feinstein and R. Picciotto (eds) *Evaluation and Poverty Reduction*. Washington, DC: World Bank. pp. 103-111.

Wenger, E. (1998) 'Communities of practice: learning, meaning and identity', *Journal of Mathematics Teacher Education*, 6(2): 185–6.

Wenger, E. (2002) *Communities of Practice. Learning, Meaning, and Identity*. Cambridge: Cambridge University Press.

West, M.A. (1990) 'The social psychology of innovation in groups', in M.A. West and J.L. Farr (eds) *Innovation and Creativity in Work: Psychological and Organisational Strategies*. Chichester: Wiley. pp. 309–34.

West, M.A., Eckert, R., Steward, K. and Pasmore, B. (2014) *Developing Collective Leadership for Health Care*. London: The King's Fund.

White, H. (2009) *Theory-based Impact Evaluation: Principles and Practice. Working Paper 3*. New Delhi: International Initiative for Impact Evaluation.

White, J. (1995) 'Patterns of knowing: review, critique and update', *Advances in Nursing Science*, 17(4): 73–86.

Wildridge, V. and Bell, L. (2002) 'How CLIP became ECLIPSE: a mnemonic to assist in search-ing for health policy/management information', *Health Information and Libraries Journal*, 19(2): 113–15.

Wilkinson, J., Powell, A. and Davies, H. (2011) 'Are clinicians engaged in quality improvement?', The Health Foundation, May.

Williamson, T., Rawle, A., Bacon, E., et al. (2006) *An Evaluation of a Nurse Led Unit: An Action Research Study*. Manchester: University of Salford, Monograph. https://usir.salford.ac.uk/id/eprint/12868/.

Willis Commission (2012) *Quality with Compassion: The Future of Nursing Education. Report of the Willis Commission on Nursing Education*. London: The Royal College of Nursing.

Wilson, M. & Greenhill, A. (2004) *Theory and Action for Emancipation: Elements of a Critical Realist Approach*. Manchester School of Management: UMIST.

Woodbridge, K. and Fulford, K.W.M. (2004) *Whose Values: A Workbook for Values-based Practice in Mental Health Care*. London: Sainsbury Centre for Mental Health.

Wye, L. & McClenahan, J. (2000) *Getting Better With Evidence: Experiences Of Putting Evidence Into Practice*. London: Kings Fund Publishing.

Wynants, L., Van Calster, B., Collins, G.S., Riley, R.D., Heinze, G., Schuit, E., Bonten, M.M.J., Dahly, D.L., Damen, J.A.A., Debray, T.P.A., de Jong, V.M.T., De Vos, M., Dhiman, P., Haller, M.C., Harhay, M.O., Henckaerts, L., Heus, P., Kammer, M., Kreuzberger, N., Lohmann, A., Luijken, K., Ma, J., Martin, G.P., McLernon, D.J., Andaur Navarro, C.L., Reitsma, J.B., Sergeant, J.C., Shi, C., Skoetz, N., Smits, L.J.M., Snell, K.I.E., Sperrin, M., Spijker, R., Steyerberg, E.W., Takada, T., Tzoulaki, I., van Kuijk, S.M.J., van Bussel, B., van der Horst, I.C.C., van Royen, F.S., Verbakel, J.Y., Wallisch, C., Wilkinson, J., Wolff, R., Hooft, L., Moons, K.G.M. and van Smeden, M. (2020) 'Prediction models for diagnosis and prognosis of Covid-19: systematic review and critical appraisal', *BMJ*, 369: m1328. https://doi.org/10.1136/bmj.m1328

Xavier, M.L., Carvalho, M.E.B de, Goncalves, M.B. dos S., Rego, A.S., Sanchez, M.C.O., Pimentel, M.R.A.R. and Chrizostimo, M.M. (2021) 'The use of photography as a research source on historical studies on nursing', *Research, Society and Development*, 10(5): 1–13.

Yin, R.K. (2018) *Case Study Research and Applications: Design and Methods* (6th edn). Thousand Oaks, CA: Sage.

Zellner, K., Boerst, C.J. and Tabb, W. (2007) 'Statistics used in current nursing research', *Journal of Nurse Education*, 46(2): 55–9.

Zieber, M. and Wojtowicz, D. (2019) 'To dwell within: bridging the theory–practice gap', *Nursing Philosophy*, December.

Index

Page numbers in *italics* refer to figures and tables, and those in **bold** indicate boxes.